Future Proof Your Skin™

*Slow down your biological clock
by changing the way you eat*

**DR STEFANIE WILLIAMS, MD,
Dermatologist**

DISCLAIMER

The recommendations outlined in this book are personal opinions of the author. None of the information included here or on our website should be construed as an attempt to offer medical advice. It is meant to be of a general educational nature and is not a substitute for the advice of your own doctor or physician.

We cannot take any responsibility for the consequences of attempts to adopt any of the recommendations presented in this book or on any featured website. We will not be liable for any damages arising from the use of this book or any website that we refer to.

No warranty is made that any of this information is accurate or up-to-date. Although the author has made every effort to ensure that the information in this book was correct at the time of writing, we do not assume and hereby disclaim any liability caused by errors or omissions, whether such errors or omissions result from negligence, accident or any other cause. All warranties are disclaimed, express and implied.

Evidence is naturally constantly evolving, especially in this area, so before you set out to follow any of our recommendations, please do your own research and, most importantly, speak to your doctor.

Please note that the method of eating described in this book is a system for adults and, for various reasons, is not designed for children.

Mention of specific companies, organizations or authorities in this book or our website does not imply endorsement by the author, nor does mention of specific companies, organizations or authorities imply that they endorse this book or its author.

EUDELO PUBLISHING

Forewords

As a registered dietician and book author, I follow a lot of what is written on nutrition for the general public. Unfortunately, I have found that most of what doctors and nutritionists are advising is appallingly out of touch with the newest scientific evidence. People are inexcusably led to hang on to dietary advice, which is completely out of date. But that's not surprising; as when you look at how our nutritional guidelines have been developed, a lot of it seems to be based more on ego and political considerations than science.

I am thrilled to see a forward-thinking professional like Dr Stefanie Williams take on dated doctrines and challenge the current sticking points in nutrition. Here is a liberating new way of eating for life, to improve health, longevity and your skin. Until hearing confirmation from a medical doctor, people find it hard to accept fundamental changes. People also don't understand why the government isn't providing the right advice. Dr Stefanie's guidance will change that. It's about time!

As Dr Stefanie is not only a medical doctor, but also a dermatologist, you will hear from the most authoritative source regarding what you should and should not be eating in order to slow down your internal aging process. I absolutely love this book and I am sure you will as well.

Aglaée Jacob, MS, RD, CDE
Registered Dietitian

Dr Stefanie Williams has proven herself as an inspirational doctor and powerful leader with this truly groundbreaking book. She is a dermatologist at the forefront of her field and guides you to achieve beautiful skin and longevity using her remarkable plan. It's not only about looking younger, but actually being younger on a biological level!

Dr Stefanie's book is extremely well referenced with scientific literature. It kept me captivated and intrigued from the first to the last page. This book is not only aimed at women; it genuinely captured my interest as a man as to how to stay vital and looking good.

This is an absolute must-read. It is bursting with trade secrets and insider information you wouldn't be able to find anywhere else. It will inspire you to take action now and change your life and your skin for the better!

Raymond Aaron
New York Times Bestselling Author

INTRODUCTION

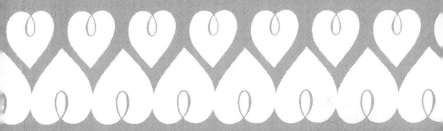

Follow me into the rabbit hole

This book will change your life as it has changed mine. It reveals previously unknown secrets to dramatically slow down your biological clock, not only in your skin, but in your entire body. I have been painstakingly researching the scientific literature on how to slow down the aging process at a cellular level for many years. Once I assembled a comprehensive system based on the outcomes of my research, I started changing my lifestyle accordingly. After only a few months, I started seeing impressive changes and can now honestly say that I have never felt better in my life. After being repeatedly asked to reveal my anti-aging secrets, I decided to share my knowledge and experience in this book. I have called my system the 'Future Food Plan™' because it is all about future proofing your skin and future proofing your entire body and mind.

This book is not only about keeping your skin looking healthy and beautiful, but also about how to stay young within. It is about extending life span while feeling fit, well and happy because what is the use of having the most amazing skin if you die of a heart attack or cancer at the age of 55? These diseases are the number one killers in the Western world. However, it is estimated that 30 to 40% of all cancers and an even higher percentage of diabetes and cardiovascular disease could be prevented by lifestyle and dietary measures alone (Donaldson et al. Nutr J. 2004)!

The underlying goal of my Future Food Plan™ is therefore to take optimal health into high age. For me, this equals true 'anti-aging'! Having beautiful, young looking skin is simply a great side effect of this. The Future Food Plan™ not only slows down the clock, but also has astounding 'side effects' including finding your optimal weight (without even trying) and cutting the risk of many modern diseases, including diabetes, cancer and heart disease. The Future Food Plan™ is also a great dietary strategy for people with inflammatory skin conditions such as acne.

While some people may be genetically lucky and, seemingly without any effort, be able to maintain healthy, young looking skin into high age, most of us are not that fortunate. However, in this book, I will share the secret of why we are not just a 'slave to our genes', but how you can actively influence them. You have to understand that genes merely express tendencies and that they are affected by our lifestyle. Newest research from the area of epigenetics has confirmed that genes do not behave like a light switch (i.e. either on or off, present or absent), but more like a light dimmer. The authors of *The Immortality Edge* state that only 30% of what happens to us is determined by our genes (i.e. inheritance), and that the other 70% can be attributed to our environment and how well we maintain ourselves (Fossel et al. John Wiley & Sons Inc. 2011). Renowned longevity researcher, Ray Kurzweil, says that only 20% is based on genetic influence and that 80% is due to the lifestyle choices we make every day (Kurzweil et al. Rodale. 2009).

The aim of the Future Food Plan™ is to trigger an ideal gene expression of your individual genetic potential. You will achieve this by inducing a beneficial hormonal and metabolic balance in your body and skin which, in turn, will support longevity, and beautiful, healthy, young looking skin. I want you to become biologically younger from within, not just show fewer lines and wrinkles on the surface.

Perceived age has scientifically been proven to be a good estimate of general health (Noordam et al. Age (Dordr). 2013). It has also been shown that the younger we look, the more likely we are to live a long life (Gunn et al. J Gerontol A Biol Sci Med Sci. 2013). The desire to look young must thus have deep evolutionary roots, as scientific evidence confirms a connection between inner health and outer youthfulness. With the Future Food Plan™ you will be improving both.

However, be aware that the Future Food Plan™ is not a 'miracle cure'; it is a way of life. You will change the way you eat for good and the more committed you are, the better the results.

I can promise that what you learn in this book will challenge long-held beliefs and transform your view of what comprises a 'healthy' lifestyle. I will introduce you to completely new concepts, such as why the current 'healthy' eating advice actually makes you age quicker. A great deal of the information discussed here is derived from cutting-edge scientific evidence. We all know that information challenging long-held beliefs is often controversial and takes time to accept. The public and even most doctors may not be aware of this evidence yet, as it has not entered mainstream medical practice.

My advice is not to listen blindly to people stuck in conservatism or healthcare practitioners trapped in old paradigms! Personally, I wouldn't want to wait until society as a whole is gradually progressing towards a healthier lifestyle; it could be decades from now. I want to be at the forefront of new developments.

So, listen to my advice and the evidence behind it and then do your own research and make up your mind independently. But for now, follow me for your breathtaking journey into the rabbit hole.

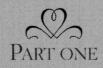

PART ONE

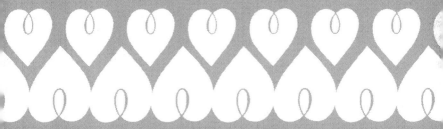

Chapter 1

Our genes and the modern world want a divorce

In order to appreciate the reasoning behind the Future Food Plan™, it is essential to understand what makes us age in the first place. What happens on a cellular level when we age? What accelerates these processes and, just as importantly, what slows them down?

Biological aging or senescence (from the Latin senescere 'to grow old') is the internal process by which our body changes, ultimately resulting in functional deterioration. Senescent cells make us look wrinkly, withered and old, and lead to degenerative diseases of aging. While the inevitable outcome of senescence is death, at least for the moment, we can significantly slow down the cellular aging process with simple lifestyle changes.

Everyone has a genetic age potential. However, things we do or are unknowingly exposed to on a daily basis speed up the aging process and significantly diminish the chance of reaching our full age potential. In addition, we will also age much less 'successfully'. Rather than remaining fit and well into high age, we will become frail, dependent and miserable. Nobody wants that.

Of course, even when following the Future Food Plan™ to the letter, there is no guarantee that we will live to be 150. As far as I know we may be run over by a bus tomorrow. But we certainly give it our very best shot! By following the Future Food Plan™, we create as perfect conditions as possible for our body and our skin, not only living longer and looking beautiful along the way, but also staying healthy, fit and independent into high age.

Exponential growth in anti-aging research
And there is more exciting news! By helping to extend our life span with the Future Food Plan™, we will be bridging over to a time when science will have advanced greatly and the potential to prolong life will have increased exponentially. I am delighted to tell you that today's prominent aging researchers believe that, if we manage to slow down the aging process naturally with lifestyle changes, we may then benefit from entering into a hotly anticipated time when science will have managed to extend lifespan to unthinkable levels!

According to Dr Aubrey De Grey, a renowned researcher in the science of aging: "The first human beings who will live to 1000 years old have probably already been born." So with that in mind, we need to ensure that we are in perfect shape when entering those exciting times. And it would be quite nice to know that we won't look 1000 years old when we get there.

So let's start by investigating why life today does not do us any favors, but actually makes us (unnecessarily!) age at lightning speed. Unfortunately, today's environment and lifestyle are not aligned with our 'hard-wiring', i.e. our genes. This leads to acceleration of the aging process and development of the many 'modern' diseases unheard of in the past.

Genetically, we still have an almost identical profile to our cave-dwelling ancestors in the Paleolithic age, i.e. caveman and cavewoman. However, our environment and lifestyle have changed dramatically, leaving us ill equipped to live in today's modern world. Our genetic heritage works against us even more when we start to reach 'middle' age, i.e. from our thirties or forties, but more about that later. The good news is that we can turn this dismal situation around with simple lifestyle changes. But before I explain how, let's have a look at why our cells age. It will help our understanding the individual steps of the Future Food Plan™.

Telomeres as markers of biological age

Aging is not a single process. It is a complex combination of different processes taking place in and around our cells at the same time. One critical event happening in every single cell of our body when we age is the shortening of our telomeres. These are the end bits of our chromosomes (the chromosomes code our genetic information in the form of DNA). Telomeres maintain the integrity and stability of our genetic material by protecting our chromosomes, a bit like the firm plastic end on a shoelace. Every time a cell divides, our chromosomes naturally erode a little and become shorter. However, it is crucial that the genetic information in our chromosomes remains fully intact in order to avoid genetic defects. So, to keep this important information safe, nature has stuck these little telomeres on to the end of our chromosomes. With every cell division, our telomeres take the brunt and shorten a little in order to protect the vital genetic information between them. This 'sacrifice' means that the functional part of our chromosome can be safely replicated without being damaged. However, once the telomeres are used up, that's the end of that particular cell.

> **Chromosomes:** Structures containing genes, the units responsible for transmission of our hereditary characteristics.
>
> **DNA:** Deoxyribonucleic acid, the main constituent of chromosomes in all organisms.
>
> **Telomeres:** Occur at the end of a chromosome, derived from the Greek words 'telos' meaning end and 'meros' meaning part.

Telomere length therefore displays our true biological cell age as opposed to mere chronological age. Fascinatingly, we can measure our telomere lengths with a simple blood test. In co-operation with our expert partner laboratory, we offer this service in our clinic. While I was initially doubtful about the benefit of knowing, I now honestly believe that finding out your true biological age is invaluable. If your biological age is found to be younger than your passport age, you will obviously be delighted and spurred on to continue your good work. If, however, your biological age is revealed to be 20 years older than the number of candles on your last cake (yes, that really can happen), there is no better motivation to change your lifestyle and do everything you can to slow down this process. And that's all this book is about.

So what can happen when our telomeres become too short? Well, it's not a pretty story. Shorter telomeres are linked to increased cancer risk and even a shortened life span (Wentzensen et al. Cancer Epidemiol Biomarkers Prev. 2011; Shen et al. Cancer Res. 2007). Longer telomeres on the other hand generally correlate with a longer life. Skin cells have been described as particularly susceptible to accelerated telomere shortening because of their high proliferation rate and exposure to DNA-damaging influences such as oxidative stress (Buckingham et al. Exp Dermatol. 2011; Boukamp. Curr Mol Med. 2005).

It was originally thought that there is a natural limit to how many times an individual cell can replicate. This so-called 'Hayflick limit' was introduced by Professor Leonard Hayflick at Stanford University many years ago and suggests a maximum possible human life span. It was believed that the Hayflick limit was due to telomere shortening during cell division. However, today we know that this is not completely correct as telomere shortening happens at different rates. Here is the good news – we can influence the rate of telomere shortening with our own lifestyle choices!

Telomere shortening and thus cell aging is accelerated by any sort of cellular stress. The more free radicals present in our tissues and the greater the oxidative stress our cells are exposed to, the faster our telomeres shorten. Smoking, chronic stress, high levels of blood sugar, low-grade inflammation and obesity have also all been linked to telomere shortening (Epel et al. Psychoneuroendocrinology. 2006). With the Future Food Plan™, we optimize negative influences leading to accelerated telomere shortening, thus slowing down the rate at which our cells age. So now we know that we can slow down the process of telomere shortening with lifestyle changes. But there is more fascinating news – telomeres can grow longer again. If you slow down telomere shortening, you slow down aging, but if you manage to actually lengthen telomeres, you reverse aging in those cells! This latter process is achieved with the help of an enzyme called telomerase. Unfortunately, the ability to produce this enzyme is switched off in most of our cells under normal conditions, but it is possible to activate it.

Dr Dean Ornish published a study confirming that changes in nutrition and lifestyle can cause the expression of over 500 genes to change in just three months (Ornish et al. Proc Natl Acad Sci U S A. 2008). In a second study, the authors showed that lifestyle changes can also induce telomerase production (Ornish et al. Lancet Oncol. 2008). Although I don't agree with all his recommendations, the studies clearly show that lifestyle intervention is able to influence our genes as well as improve telomere length. The importance of this research was emphasized when the 2009 Nobel Prize for Medicine was awarded to three scientists for their work on telomerase activity (Ventegodt et al. Int J Adolesc Med Health. 2012; Falus et al. Orv Hetil. 2010).

Telomere biology also ties in perfectly with the other mechanisms of aging, including oxidative damage, glycation, abnormal methylation and hormonal imbalance or deterioration. These all sound like complex terms and I do talk more about them later but, in the meantime, it is important to understand that, at a cellular level, they all contribute significantly to aging and create havoc not only in our skin but in our entire body. They were 'designed' by nature to perform specific, useful functions, but today's modern lifestyle can lead them to turn on us and become more harmful than useful. Let's have a look at these mechanisms in more detail.

Oxidative stress

Free radicals are unstable molecules that steal electrons from other molecules in our body, including proteins, lipids and even our DNA, i.e. the molecule that encodes our genetic information. Examples include reactive oxygen species (ROS) and reactive nitrogen species (RNS).

Free radicals: Unstable molecules that steal electrons from other molecules in our body.

Oxidative stress: The result of an imbalance between the production of free radicals and a cell's ability to detoxify the products it creates or repair the damage they cause.

Glycation: When sugar molecules attach themselves to other molecules, for example proteins.

Advanced Glycation End products (AGEs): Formed when sugar molecules cross-link with a protein, for example collagen in the skin, and affect the protein's function.

Methylation: The process where a methyl group (CH_3) attaches itself to other molecules such as DNA. Normal methylation is a useful mechanism; abnormal methylation can increase your risk of certain diseases, including cancer.

Every cell in our body generates free radicals. They are a product of routine metabolic processes that take place every second of every day. They are usually neutralized by agents called antioxidants and so the balance of free radical formation and neutralization is maintained. However, with today's lifestyle, the generation of free radicals is often significantly amplified. Smoking, sun exposure, pollution, toxins, stress and the wrong type of diet can all lead to increased production of free radicals. Our natural antioxidant pool can't cope with the increased demand and becomes exhausted, upsetting the delicate balance. This misbalance is known as oxidative stress and the inevitable consequence is damage to cellular structures.

Oxidative stress and inadequate clearance of material damaged in the process is now acknowledged as a key mechanism in aging, not only in our skin, but in all major systems of our body. Oxidative stress can even cause mutations in our DNA and lead to cancer. One of the main aims of any anti-aging strategy, therefore, should be to reduce free radical production and increase antioxidant levels in your body. Studies have confirmed that good dietary habits are a major determinant of our body's antioxidant status and oxidative stress level (Anlasik et al. Br J Nutr. 2005; Polidori et al. J Alzheimers Dis. 2009). With simple changes to the way we eat, the Future Food Plan™ supports this balance naturally. We can also measure your antioxidant status with a blood test.

Glycation
Glycation is also a very important mechanism of aging (Avery et al. Pathol Biol [Paris]. 2006). It refers to the process where sugar molecules attach themselves to other molecules in our body, for example proteins. In the skin, the sugar molecules

cross link important proteins such as collagen, to form Advanced Glycation End products (AGEs). This process renders the cross-linked collagen inferior and leads to inflammation. Naturally, the more sugar circulating in our blood the more sugar molecules there are available to attach themselves to proteins. Preformed AGEs are also present in many of the foods we consume. The levels depend on the type of food and how it is prepared and I talk more about that later.

Our personal glycation levels can be measured using a simple blood test – Hemoglobin A1c (Hb A1c). It tells you how much glycation has been taking place in your cells over the past few months. Fructosamine testing can also give you that information, but looks at a shorter time frame (past few weeks rather than months). We offer both tests in our clinic; it is a powerful piece of information if you want to future proof yourself. The Future Food Plan™ will significantly reduce harmful glycation processes and AGE levels not only in your skin, but your entire body.

Inflammation

Originally, acute inflammation was a beneficial process for our body. The symptoms of swelling, redness, warmth and pain were signs of healing trauma and fighting infections in a world without antibiotics. However, too much of a good thing can become a bad thing and that's clearly the case with inflammation. In today's world, chronic stress, supposedly healthy diets and other modern lifestyle habits lead to a low-grade, chronic inflammation. This invisible form of inflammation smolders silently in our body, often for decades without obvious symptoms. However, all along it accelerates aging.

There is a strong association between chronic low-grade inflammatory activity and long-term tissue damage and aging, not only in our skin, but throughout our entire body. Inflammation is also involved in many modern diseases such as heart disease and metabolic syndrome (a combination of diabetes, high blood pressure, high blood lipids and obesity that increases your risk of heart attack or stroke). In summary, chronic inflammation makes us age quicker and die younger and therefore should be reduced at all costs.

A number of factors can contribute to chronic inflammation. These include high blood sugar and insulin levels and oxidative stress. It is possible to measure the general level of inflammation in our body with a blood test called hsCRP (high sensitivity C-reactive protein). In the absence of infection or inflammatory conditions such as arthritis, which cause the CRP level to rise, your CRP level should be low. Interestingly, a sedentary lifestyle, smoking and poor sleep have also been found to raise your CRP level (Kurzweil. Rodale. 2009). Again, we offer CRP measurements in our clinic.

Abnormal Methylation
Methylation is a process where a methyl group (i.e. one carbon atom bonds with three hydrogen atoms = CH_3) attaches itself to other organic molecules including our DNA. It is a very useful mechanism, as it helps to stabilize telomeres and regulate the epigenetic expression of genes. Epigenetics is a fascinating new area of research – the study of the biological processes that cause changes in our gene expression without altering the underlying DNA sequence, i.e. the genes themselves. Epigenetics has revealed that our body is able to

repress or activate certain genes. The prefix 'epi' in epigenetics comes from the Greek word for 'over' or 'above'.

Methylation is an example of a mechanism where lifestyle factors can change the expression of our inherited genes. This is an amazing fact in itself – we have power, we can influence our genes! Even more extraordinary is that some epigenetic changes to the genome have even been shown to pass down to the next generation (Spector. W&N. 2012)! This all happens without any change to the underlying DNA sequence. We simply cause our genes to behave (or 'express themselves') differently. This is an example of how environmental influences can silence 'bad genes' and allow 'good genes' to be read instead.

So, when methylation works well, it is a great process. However, a proportion of the population have an abnormal methylation, which can lead to development of cardiovascular disease and cancer, including the deadliest form of skin cancer, melanoma (Schinke et al. Melanoma Res. 2010; Li et al. World J Gastroenterol. 2012). One way of measuring your methylation status is to measure the level of homocysteine in your blood, a molecule which accumulates if you have abnormal methylation.

DNA mutations

Although our genes (and the DNA sequence they contain) are inherited from our parents, there are occasions where the DNA sequence may be damaged and changed permanently, leading to a gene mutation. Environmental influences have the potential to cause DNA damage and mutations and, unfortunately, the older we get, the more DNA damage we accumulate. Not all mutations are bad, but there is a possibility that they can lead to impaired cell function and serious consequences such as the development of cancer.

Mutations are not confined to our 'normal' DNA within the cell nucleus (the control center of a cell); they also happen outside the nucleus, in our mitochondria. These tiny organelles are our cells' power houses; the place where 'fuel is burned' to generate an energy molecule called adenosine triphosphate (ATP) during 'cellular respiration'. Because the generation of ATP molecules is vital for cell functioning, mitochondria are essential to our health and longevity. Unfortunately, the energy production in our mitochondria is susceptible to free radical production and oxidative stress. The older we get the less effective our mitochondria are and the more free radicals they are likely to generate during their work. Imagine a soaring new car engine compared to an old one spitting out black smoke. Do you get the picture?

Mitochondria: Small, spherical or rod-like bodies found in the cytoplasm of cells. Resonsible for our cells' energy generation.
Organelles: Literally, 'little organs' that perform special functions in the cell.
Cellular respiration: A series of metabolic processes in a cell, which generate biochemical energy in the form of adenosine triphosphate (ATP).

Intriguingly, mitochondria, unlike any other cell organelle, have their own DNA – called mtDNA. It is completely separate from the cell nucleus, where our main DNA lives. Its position at the center of cell power generation means that mtDNA is particularly vulnerable to free radical production during cellular respiration. The DNA repair mechanisms of mitochondria are also not as effective as those in the nucleus, rendering them particularly susceptible to accumulation of DNA mutations.

So, in summary, our cells accumulate DNA mutations inside and outside the cell nucleus with age. While some of these mutations may be silent or in certain cases even beneficial, other mutations may lead to impaired function and harmful consequences such as cancer.

'Junk' in and around cells

With increasing age, our body's decreasing ability to recycle material effectively leads to a gradual buildup of damaged proteins in and around our cells. This aggregation of 'junk' material plays an important part in aging (De Grey et al. St. Martin's Griffin. 2008).

As we age, our skin is also unable to produce proteins, such as collagen and elastin, as quickly and as well as it used to. And to make matters worse, it also degrades them quicker (Mays et al. Int J Biochem Cell Biol. 1995). Certain environmental factors such as smoking and sun exposure further induce a group of enzymes called matrix-metallo-proteinases (MMPs) in our skin (Gruss et al. Lancet. 1997). One of these MMPs is collagenase, whose job it is to degrade collagen – not good news for our skin!

Hormonal balance

Hormones are our body's chemical messengers, travelling in our blood and influencing many different processes. Certain hormones released into our body are 'catabolic' (break down tissue), while others are 'anabolic' (build up tissue). When we are young, anabolic and catabolic hormones are usually perfectly balanced. However, as we age, the production of some hormones declines, while production of others increases. The resulting change to the delicate hormonal balance can lead to accelerated and premature aging. With a skin-friendly and anti-aging way of eating such as the Future Food Plan™, we can encourage the release of anabolic 'youth' hormones while moderating release of inflammatory and catabolic 'aging' hormones and help restore hormonal balance. Let's take a closer look at some of these hormones to understand the nutritional changes needed to achieve this balance.

Aging hormones

Important pro-aging hormones include the stress hormones cortisol, adrenaline and noradrenaline (I will refer to the latter two collectively as adrenaline here simply to make things easier to read). They are secreted by our adrenal glands, which sit on top of our kidneys (the name 'renal' comes from the Latin word for kidney).

For our ancestors living in a primitive world, a short burst of stress hormone release was beneficial as it optimized the fight-or-flight reaction when faced with danger, for example, escaping from a predator. During this reaction, release of stress hormones ensured that we had enough resources and ideal conditions to address this urgent threat. Our body tensed up and became very alert; our blood sugar level increased to supply energy, our heart rate accelerated and our blood pressure rose. The rate at which our blood clotted also increased so that we wouldn't bleed to death if wounded. As the extra energy provided would be burned off immediately with intense physical activity (i.e. attacking or running away), everything would return to normal quite quickly.

In today's modern world, luckily, we don't face many life-or-death situations like this. However, we are exposed to a fairly constant level of chronic, low-level stress for which there is usually no physical release. Chronic stress can lead to an elevation of cortisol and other stress hormones.

Pro-aging hormones include **stress hormones** (adrenaline, noradrenaline and cortisol) and **insulin.**

Under normal physiological circumstances, our cortisol release is high in the morning, just after getting up, and then gradually declines during the day. However, when we are chronically stressed, the cortisol level may remain high throughout the day. Not only can this lead to fatigue of the adrenal glands but excess release of cortisol creates a catabolic state, and leads to destruction of collagen in the skin and other important structures in our body. In order to slow down aging, we therefore have to minimize the release of stress hormones.

Scientists have known for a while that cortisol levels are associated with our health (Noordam et al. Psychoneuroendocrinology. 2012). However, it has now been confirmed that high levels of cortisol are also linked to our face looking older (Noordam et al. Psychoneuroendocrinology. 2012)!

Insulin, secreted in the beta cells of our pancreas (which sits just under our ribs on the left), is another major pro-aging hormone in our body. Insulin is the master hormone for regulating fat and carbohydrate metabolism. At optimal levels, insulin is our friend, clearing away excess sugar from our blood. However, when present in excess, it becomes our enemy, promoting inflammation, aging and weight gain. The latter is caused by insulin clearing away sugar from our blood stream and converting a large proportion of it into fat.

Insulin is the key to our fat cells – it is needed to unlock them and allow sugar to enter for fat conversion and storage. Insulin also signals abundance of external energy (i.e. food) to our body and suppresses breakdown of fat tissue. You can imagine it like this: when times are bad and energy is sparse, we need to start breaking down our fat to use as 'fuel'. However, in times of abundance (i.e. when we consume plenty of sugar and other carbohydrates to supply our body with energy), there is no need to start nibbling on our long-term store of fat tissue; this can be saved for times of scarcity. Not ideal if you are hoping for fat loss. But apart from insulin's anabolic effect on fat tissue, it also accelerates the aging process at a cellular level. Insulin promotes chronic, low-level inflammation, stimulates cortisol production and hinders the work of some of our 'youth hormones'.

A good sensitivity of our cells to insulin (so that our pancreas doesn't have to overproduce insulin to 'get the message through') is very important and superior insulin sensitivity is connected to familial longevity (Wijsman et al. Aging Cell. 2011).

With today's way of eating, insulin accelerates aging like no other hormone (see later); therefore we should try and moderate our insulin secretion. I am not suggesting insulin is all bad; without it we wouldn't be able to survive. But no worries, there will always be a sufficient basal insulin secretion (this in fact accounts for over 50% of our total insulin secretion), independent of carbohydrate intake (Wilcox et al. Clin Biochem Rev. 2005). We should, however, avoid the excess insulin secretion we see with today's Western diet.

Youth hormones

Now we've looked at aging hormones such as cortisol, adrenaline and insulin, it's time to talk about some 'youth' hormones. Growth hormones are important youth hormones. They perform a variety of physiological functions relating to growth and metabolism in our body. We have a number of different growth hormones and growth factors circulating at all times, including Human Growth Hormone (HGH, also known as the 'fitness hormone') and Insulin-like-Growth Factor 1 (IGF-1). Growth hormones in general are known to be anabolic type hormones.

HGH is secreted in a pulsatile manner by our pituitary gland (a pea-sized gland at the base of our brain). In turn, it stimulates the secretion of IGF-1 in our liver, which assists in many of the growth promoting actions of HGH throughout our body. As our natural level of HGH goes down with age, HGH has been named the 'youth hormone' and reduced levels are used as a marker of aging. Declining HGH levels are known to lead to a reduction in lean muscle mass and an accumulation of fat with increasing age. It has also been described as partly responsible for the thinning of our skin that occurs in old age (Rudman et al. N Engl J Med. 1990). Higher IGF-1 levels have been shown to be connected to reduced skin wrinkling (Noordam et al. Br J Dermatol. 2013).

> **Youth promoting hormones** include **growth hormones,** for example Human Growth Hormone (HGH, also known as the 'fitness hormone'); **sex hormones** such as estrogen, progesterone, DHEA and testosterone and **melatonin,** known as the 'sleep hormone'.

So, it sounds as if high levels of growth hormones can only be a good thing when keeping your skin and body in top shape, right? In fact, that's why some well-meaning anti-aging practitioners started to inject growth hormone to encourage skin and body rejuvenation in their patients. However, the latest research shows that the situation is unfortunately not that straightforward. While growth hormones certainly stimulate the cell and tissue growth, they have also been shown to reduce a tissue's resistance to oxidative stress, an effect that generally shortens the life span of an organism and is a risk factor for certain cancers, including breast, colon and prostate cancer.

And sure enough, accumulating evidence now suggests that the HGH/IGF-1 axis plays an important role in aging and positive effects on body composition and skin quality may come at a significant cost in terms of longevity and susceptibility to age-related diseases (Oh et al. Clin Chim Acta. 2012; Laron. Mech Ageing Dev. 2005; Masternak et al. Pathobiol Aging Age Relat Dis. 2012). So there seems to be a trade-off.

IGF-1 appears to generate particular concern. Lower levels of IGF-1 have been shown to improve cell repair rather than encouraging production of new cells (and burning the candle at both ends). Research has confirmed that mutant mice lacking growth hormone age slower and outlive their normal siblings by as much as 40 to 60%! This improved longevity appears to be due to multiple mechanisms including reduced oxidative damage, enhanced resistance to stress, reduced insulin levels and delayed onset of age-related disease (Bartke. Endocrinology. 2005).

In a recent study it was found that the offspring of centenarians had lower IGF-I activity compared to offspring of people who died relatively young (Vitale et al. Aging (Albany NY). 2012). Interestingly, this lower IGF-I bioactivity also correlated with improved insulin sensitivity.

Collectively, these results suggest that optimizing the HGH/IGF-1 axis to promote healthy aging is more complex than originally appreciated and requires a greater understanding of the multiple interactions. So while research in this area keeps developing, I advise against growth hormone injections until we know more. It is imperative that we optimize our growth hormone levels naturally, without the damaging consequences of increased insulin levels, amplified generation of free radicals, oxidative damage and reduced resistance to stress.

In addition to growth hormones, growth factors such as EGF (Epidermal Growth Factor), FGF (Fibroblast Growth Factor) and PDGF (Platelet-derived Growth Factor) are also present in our body. These are all proteins that stimulate the proliferation and differentiation of cells and induce protein synthesis. They act as signaling molecules between cells and are produced locally throughout the body.

Sex hormones
Sex hormones such as estrogen, progesterone and testosterone have a profound influence on our skin and can also be considered as youth-promoting hormones.

Estrogens are known to help prevent skin aging in women, especially in those who are post-menopausal. They improve female collagen production, skin thickness, texture, hydration, and wound healing. Estrogen has also been shown to promote telomerase activity and protect against telomere shortening (Emmerson et al. Biogerontology. 2012). Around the age of 50 years, as women enter the menopause (which simply means cessation of menstruation), our estrogen and progesterone levels drop dramatically, an event which plays a major role in the aging process. There is loss of bone volume, muscle mass, and also loss of skin thickness and function. Can you believe that women lose a staggering 30% of their skin's collagen content in the first five years after menopause? Furthermore, low estrogen levels accompanying the menopause accelerate the damaging effects of environmental (external) aging.

Beneficial effects of hormone replacement therapy (HRT) on skin aging have been well documented but, understandably, HRT cannot be recommended solely to prevent skin aging in post-menopausal women (Savvas et al. Br J Obstet Gynaecol. 1993; Studd et al. Menopause Int. 2010; Verdier-Sévrain et al. Climacteric. 2007). Topical estrogen application has been shown to be beneficial in post-menopausal skin. However, this type of skincare would need to be prescribed and supervised by an experienced doctor as, depending on the concentration, there may be some systemic absorption of the hormone into the blood stream.

Aging in men is also associated with a progressive decline in the production of sex hormones such as testosterone (a phase known as andropause). Testosterone is a natural anabolic hormone, which preserves muscle and bone mass. Men with declining levels of testosterone experience loss of muscle and bone mass, fat gain (especially around the middle) and thinning of the skin. Although it is classed as a male hormone, women also secrete testosterone, albeit at much lower levels. Sufficient testosterone levels are not only crucial for male health, but also for female well-being and vitality.

DHEA (dehydroepiandrosterone) is a less well-known sex hormone. It is also considered a 'youth hormone' as its level declines dramatically with increasing age (von Mühlen et al. Contemp Clin Trials. 2007). DHEA is a precursor of other sex hormones including testosterone and possesses anti-inflammatory activity. It lowers the level of pro-inflammatory cytokines and enhances immune functions (Wang et al. Atherosclerosis. 2011; von Mühlen et al. Contemp Clin Trials. 2007). Epidemiological evidence suggests that DHEA may also have a protective effect against heart disease, obesity and diabetes (von Mühlen et al. Contemp Clin Trials. 2007) and, when applied topically, it has been shown to increase collagen production and improve structural organization of the dermis, the crucial middle layer of our skin, where most of our skin's collagen lives (Calvo et al. J Steroid Biochem Mol Biol. 2008).

Melatonin

Melatonin is a hormone derived from serotonin produced in the pineal gland (a tiny, pine cone shaped gland in the midline of our brain). It is known as the 'sleep hormone', but I would also class it as one of our 'youth hormones', as it has many positive effects on our skin.

Our melatonin level starts to rise in the evening and peaks around midnight before slowly declining again. The natural daily melatonin rhythm is triggered by changes of light and darkness. Melatonin is important for restorative sleep, which is crucial for skin and tissue repair. It also is a powerful natural antioxidant and melatonin receptors are expressed in many skin cell types. Interestingly, melatonin has been shown to protect our skin from the sun's damaging effects and counteract mitochondrial and DNA damage (Kleszczynski et al. Dermatoendocrinol. 2012). Unfortunately, our melatonin level declines with age, just like so many other 'skin friendly' hormones (Zouboulis. Hautarzt. 2003).

In summary, if we want to age successfully and maintain youthful looking skin, it is vital to maintain a balanced hormone profile, i.e. support the release of 'youth hormones' and moderate the release of 'aging hormones' in a natural and safe way.

The guiding principles of the Future Food Plan™ are to minimize oxidative stress, inflammation, glycation, abnormal methylation and telomere shortening, while positively influencing your hormonal homeostasis.

CHAPTER 2

Why skinny is out

Congratulations for making it through the last chapter with all the detailed background on the mechanisms of aging. In the following chapters, it will become obvious why this background information is crucial to understanding the components of the Future Food Plan™. You are now on your way to discover my insider tricks to slow down the aging process in your body and future proof your skin. However, before we start going into practical instructions, let's have a look at another area that has a major impact on aging; one that is not very well known at all.

With growing pervasiveness of the media, women and men of all ages are bombarded with images that glorify and link self-worth to being skinny. We are confronted with under-nourished looking models and celebrities on a daily basis and are encouraged to aim for this body shape as our ideal. The extent of this problem is confirmed by an American study revealing that more than 80% of college students diet no matter how much they weigh (Malinauskas et al. Nutr J. 2006).

Nowadays, there is so much focus on body weight and shape that it is difficult to remain objective and discuss the topic on a non-emotional level. However, let's step back and review the scientific facts. You will be surprised how much it ties in with anti-aging.

There is no doubt that malnutrition and being underweight makes our skin age quicker. Low body weight has been linked to low estrogen and DHEA levels (two of our 'youth hormones') and high cortisol levels (one of the terribly aging stress hormones) (Bates et al. Clin Obstet Gynecol. 1985; Gibbs et al. Int J Sport Nutr Exerc Metab. 2011; Howgate et al. Osteoporos Int. 2013). Low estrogen and high cortisol levels are established factors involved in the acceleration of skin aging. So for the sake of long-term skin health and vitality, it is important not to let our body weight fall below the 'normal' range, usually measured using body mass index (BMI). This is a simple way of judging if our body weight is appropriate for our height. The actual calculation is your weight (in kilograms) divided by your height (in meters) squared. However, it's much easier to go onto the internet and search for 'BMI calculator' (there are many different ones, most of which are free to use), which will calculate your BMI instantaneously. For most adults, a 'normal', healthy BMI is in the range of 18.5 to 24.9.

Under-eating AND over-exercising with extended cardio or other endurance sports is even worse! This lethal combination increases our levels of cortisol and adrenaline (the catabolic, 'using-up' stress hormones) and causes our body to 'eat itself' from within. Also, when the levels of these hormones are too high, our body will not receive the important hormonal command to regenerate itself, because our hormonal balance is completely out of sync and skewed towards breaking-down rather than building-up tissue. We will also not have enough of the essential building materials to regenerate. I see this in clinic regularly: people who consume extremely low-fat foods, essentially just eating vegetables, fruit and whole grains all day long, and then doing cardio exercise like running for a couple of hours each day. They feel that they are living a very 'clean' and healthy life, but this is far from the truth. This lifestyle does not do our skin any favors at all and will make us age at lightning speed.

Body Mass Index: A method of calculating whether your weight is appropriate for your height: $\dfrac{\text{weight (kg)}}{\text{height (m}^2)}$

Just to be clear, I am not advocating being a couch potato and not doing any exercise at all, as a sedentary lifestyle clearly has a negative impact on health and longevity (and has also been shown to shorten telomeres by the way). However, it's over-exercising with cardio and endurance sports that prematurely ages our skin and our body, but that's a topic for another book ...

I imagine finding out that being too skinny is neither good for your long-term skin health nor general health may be a relief for some readers. It is important to free yourself from society's pressure to try and lose weight if your BMI is already considered 'normal'!

However, now let's look at the other side of the equation. Sorry to be the bearer of bad news here but what you probably do not realize is that your skin not only ages more quickly if you are fashionably skinny, but also if you are overweight. Fat cells (adipocytes) shockingly have been revealed to secrete a whole range of pro-inflammatory cytokines and chemokines, which contribute to chronic low-level inflammation (Gouranton et al. J Nutr Biochem. 2011)! I am sure you remember that chronic inflammation is a very important aging factor and should be minimized.

If you are overweight, you may not notice your lines and wrinkles as much at the beginning, because they are 'padded' out with fat. But your skin is aging prematurely at an impressive rate at cellular level due to low-grade inflammatory processes. Obese people have been shown to have a higher rate of oxidative stress in their entire body. To make matters worse, scientific studies have found that the more fat we have in our body the lower our level of human growth hormone (HGH), one of our natural 'youth hormones'.

Your aim should be to have a body weight within the healthy BMI range of 18.5 – 24.9 (ideally somewhere in the middle), as both under-eating and excessive food intake impair skin function and regeneration (Piccardi et al. Dermatoendocrinol. 2009). So, if you are already within this healthy range, please don't fret about wanting to lose weight, this can actually do more harm than good. You are fine and should stop worrying. Let me repeat that – you are absolutely 100% fine! Skinny is out – healthy is in. It is time to finally accept your 'natural' weight, even if it may not be your ideal 'standing-naked-in-front-of-a-full-length-mirror-weight'. What I call 'natural' weight is the healthy body weight that we tend to fluctuate towards over time. This is who you are and it is important that you accept it.

Let me tell you a quick story. The other day I found one of my old hand-written diaries from my mid-twenties when I cleared out the attic. I started reading (cringing as you can imagine and fighting to stop myself from burning it there and then) and it really struck me how much I fussed about my weight. I was a perfectly healthy body weight, but I was constantly trying to lose weight. My diary also revealed something truly shocking that I had completely forgotten about, but more of that later. Winding forward a good decade or so, I can tell you that I did end up a little over-weight after having my three children. Have a look at www.FutureProofYourSkin.com if you want to see a photo of me from that time – you will be surprised!

However, since starting my skin health and longevity eating plan, that extra weight just fell off over time (at the time without any exercise I have to admit). I am now right in the middle of the healthy BMI range. And guess what? When I compared my body weight today with the one mentioned in my old diary, I was surprised to find out that the two are not all that different. All thanks to the Future Food Plan™.

So this is my 'natural' weight; the weight I tend to come back to when eating well. I am fully aware that I wouldn't make a living as a swimwear model but, in contrast to my twenties,

I am now happy with my weight. I know it will help me try and achieve a long and healthy life. I can also honestly say that I never felt better than now. My skin looks good and I feel great overall, without following any of that low-fat nonsense advice, but more about that later. Read on to find out why low-fat diets actually make us age rapidly!

So now is the time to stop comparing yourself to skinnier friends or people in magazines. Your natural weight may be slightly higher than you would hope for in an ideal world, but as long as it's within the healthy BMI range, there is no need to change it. However, if you are above or below the healthy range and are committed to future proofing not only your skin, but your entire body, I strongly encourage you to try and move back into that range.

Now, let me tell you something about my husband, Jay. You often hear people who are slightly above the healthy BMI range say that the BMI system is flawed. The reason usually quoted is that it does not cater for people with higher muscle mass. In fact, my own husband was one of these doubters. He kept telling me that the BMI is not applicable to him and that he is certainly not overweight – it's all muscle or so he claimed. One day, I bought some special bathroom scales, which measure your actual muscle proportion. It turned that his muscle mass was quite average and certainly did not mean that the BMI was not relevant to him. This revelation made him gradually adapt to the Future Food Plan™ way of eating and I am delighted to say that after losing more than 10kg (22 pounds) effortlessly, he has now reached his natural weight and tells me he has never felt better. He reports feeling younger now in his forties than he did in his thirties and that's despite the fact that he didn't even feel there was a problem before. You know what, I am going to also try and find a before-after photograph of Jay and put it on www.Future-ProofYourSkin.com. Hopefully he won't kill me for that, or worse, divorce me ...

Anyway, our personal stories confirm that following the Future Food Plan™ way of eating not only has anti-aging benefits, but also makes you feel amazing. It also helps you gradually achieve your natural weight, effortlessly and safely, without any calorie counting, hunger pangs or cravings. So let's talk specifics now and dive straight into the first step of the Future Food Plan™.

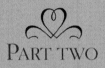

PART TWO

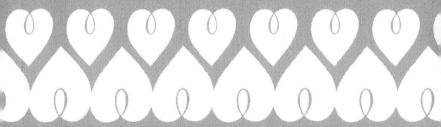

CHAPTER 3

Aging in cube form

Well done for completing the full theoretical background about aging. You now know what makes us age, but you don't yet know what to do to protect against it. So let's start with the first practical step of the Future Food Plan™. What you eat and drink on a daily basis has a major impact on your biological clock. You may think you already know what you are supposed to eat and what a healthy diet looks like but, believe me, you are in for a shock. What is commonly assumed to be a healthy diet can make us age at lightning speed if we are not careful. Unfortunately, there is a lot of misleading information out there (even from so-called 'experts') with regards to the best type of diet for your skin and overall health and longevity. For example, the officially recommended 'food pyramid', with its low-fat obsession and massive foundation of grain-based, starchy foods such as bread, pasta and potatoes, has not only led our society to become overweight and beset with diseases such as diabetes, but it doesn't do our skin any favors either.

Let me ask you a question: which external influence, other than smoking and excessive sun exposure, do you think ages your skin most? It is today's excessive sugar intake. Did you guess correctly? In a typical Western diet, we ingest way too much sugar, mainly because it is hidden in so many foods. I will give you lots of examples later, but first let me tell you why sugar is so damaging to our skin health and longevity.

Sugar

Unfortunately, we are ill equipped genetically to deal with the amount of sugar our modern diets contain. You may remember from earlier that I highlighted how, although our lifestyle has changed dramatically since caveman times, our genetic code has hardly changed at all. Cavemen and women didn't have much sugar in their diet. What they did eat came mainly from the occasional seasonal fruit if they were lucky, but it was less sweet and more fibrous than the fruit that we have nowadays. So our genetic make-up remains geared towards this low sugar content.

The amount of sugar we eat today is harmful for our skin and makes us age more quickly than need be. Sugar has a number of negative effects on our body. You may remember that sugars such as glucose, and even fructose (fruit sugar), can react with collagen and other important proteins in our skin to form tissue-harming cross links called Advanced Glycation End products (AGEs) (Danby. Clin Dermatol. 2010; Pageon. Pathol Biol (Paris) 2010; Schalkwijk et al. Diabetes Metab Res Rev. 2004). These cross-links prevent collagen from performing its optimal function as a major supporting structure in our skin. Glycation also causes other destructive reactions in our skin, including free radical formation, oxidative stress and inflammation, all of which accelerate aging. Each of these changes creates an environment that supports degradation of collagen and compromises integrity and regeneration of our skin. Some degree of glycation occurs all the time, and that's fine, but the extent of glycation in our skin is greatly increased by consuming a high sugar diet. We can significantly reduce the rate of glycation by reducing the amount of sugary foods we eat on a daily basis. Interestingly, glycation in our skin is also increased after excessive sun exposure (Danby. Clin Dermatol. 2010).

It is known that familial longevity is associated with better blood sugar control (Noordam et al. Age (Dordr). 2013). But let me tell you about the results of a truly groundbreaking study – hot off the press. In this study, people were asked to estimate the age of more than 600 strangers, purely by looking at their portrait photograph. The study revealed that higher blood sugar levels correlated with higher perceived ages (Noordam et al. Age (Dordr). 2013). In plain English – people with higher blood sugar look older! And this was independent of any confounding factors such as smoking status, gender and sun damage. A very powerful study indeed.

High sugar intake also leads to many 'modern' diseases such as metabolic syndrome (a combination of diabetes, obesity and high blood pressure), which puts us at greater risk of heart disease, stroke and other serious health problems. Elevated blood pressure, even if mild, has been shown to lead to so-called 'capillary rarefication' (i.e. reduced density of small blood vessels in the skin) (He et al. Hypertension. 2010), which can reduce the supply of oxygen and nutrients to the skin. It is also well recognized that people with diabetes, who suffer with elevated blood sugar levels, tend to develop age-related disorders much earlier than the general population.

And here are three more reasons to cut out sugar from our diet. Firstly, cancer cells rely heavily on sugar as their fuel for growth! By drastically reducing sugar intake we can limit the amount of energy available for cancer cells (Port et al. Curr Opin Endocrinol Diabetes Obes. 2012).

Secondly, a recent study confirmed that long-standing hyperglycemia (i.e. high blood sugar levels) impairs skin barrier function including protection against bacteria (Park et al. Exp Dermatol. 2011). The same study also confirmed accelerated skin aging in people with high blood sugar levels (Park et al. Exp Dermatol. 2011). Not surprisingly, the acceleration of skin aging processes was found to be in direct proportion to the duration of hyperglycaemia. Lastly, high blood sugar levels have been shown to have a negative influence on growth factor release such as our 'youth hormone' HGH.

Before we move on to the next topic, let me tell you what I saw in my son's school recently, yet again confirming my concerns. Walking through the school's corridors viewing the children's exhibits, I noticed a project on display about life in Hampton Court during the reign of Henry VIII . On a poster collage, I read that poor people actually lived longer than the rich at that time, as they did not have access to sugar, which was a luxury food item! On the other hand, the noble men and women living at Hampton Court enjoyed plenty of sugar. Apparently, even the plates were made out of sugar and completely edible. So, it seems this is not a new problem.

Insulin
Another reason why sugary foods are bad news for our skin is

that a rising blood sugar (glucose) level causes an immediate hike in insulin release, as it is insulin's job to swiftly clear away glucose from our blood stream. As I mentioned before, insulin is the key that unlocks certain cells such as adipocytes (fat cells) to facilitate the entry of glucose. Here, sugar is converted into fat and stored for later use as energy, as glucose itself cannot be stored in meaningful quantities. A small amount of glucose can be stored as glycogen in liver and muscle, but it is a relatively small amount compared to that converted into fat.

So, to recap, eating sugary foods causes our blood sugar level to rise, which immediately causes the release of insulin. Insulin, however, is one of the main 'aging' hormones, so not ideal if we want to slow down the aging process!

The well-organized teamwork of insulin and adipocytes converting sugar into fat allows our body to hold on to every calorie possible. This mechanism made a lot of sense for our primal ancestors, who never knew when their next meal would be. It allowed them to maintain constant access to an energy supply even if food intake wasn't regular. However, with the advent of refrigeration, supermarkets and the fact that we don't have to actively hunt for our food any longer, those of us living in the developed world hardly ever experience a shortage of food or famine. Unfortunately, our genetic hard-wiring hasn't been updated to reflect today's lifestyle and its virtually constant supply of food. As a result, insulin's originally useful effects can create profound trouble. While we wouldn't be able to survive without any insulin, today's excessive insulin release is causing major problems. Let's have a look at some of them.

The ups and downs of insulin release

Excessive insulin release has been shown to contribute to free radical generation, oxidative stress, inflammation and striking acceleration of skin aging. Together with high blood sugar levels, elevated insulin levels and inflammation also lead our platelets (the blood cells responsible for blood clotting) to become more 'sticky', thus increasing the risk of clots in our blood vessels (Vazzana et al. Thromb Res. 2012).

Insulin also interferes with other hormones. For example, it leads to a decrease in the levels of testosterone, DHEA and other anti-aging sex hormones, which are known to decline with age anyway. Insulin also increases the level of sex-hormone-binding-globulins, proteins that keep sex hormones bound and thus inactive. High insulin levels not only accelerate aging, but also lead to diabetes, inflammation, heart disease, cancer and many other 'modern' diseases.

It is interesting to note that without insulin our fat cells would stay locked and glucose would not be allowed to enter and be stored as fat. Some major rethinking is needed with regards to what is worse – a high-fat diet or a high-sugar diet. I think you know already what the answer is!

Not all the effects of insulin are so subtle. After a meal, there is an insulin spike, designed to clear away sugar from our blood stream. This clearing action means that our blood sugar level will plummet a couple of hours later, leaving us ravenous for more sugar and other carbohydrates! In people whose body uses sugar as its main energy source, which is the vast majority of people with a typical Western diet, low blood sugar also causes low energy levels and lethargy. Hypoglycemia (i.e. low blood sugar level) is also the reason we may experience light-headedness and possibly mild shaking a couple of hours after eating a sugar-loaded meal. Giving in to the renewed hunger and sugar cravings creates a vicious circle, leading to fluctuating high and low blood sugar levels throughout the day. Does being hungry two hours after breakfast and energy dips in the afternoon ring any bells?

The repeated ups and downs of glucose and insulin are very stressful for our body. It responds by releasing the 'aging' stress hormones, cortisol and adrenaline, which encourage collagen breakdown and lead to other negative consequences as we already know. Eventually, these continuous waves of sugar intake, blood sugar spikes and insulin hikes make our cells less responsive to insulin. It's a bit like shouting at your kids all the time. After a while, they will stop responding due to the constant 'white-noise' of a raised voice. If, however, you usually talk to your children with a calm voice, a sudden raise will achieve a much better response. This is the same with insulin: if our body is bombarded with high insulin levels all the time, our cells turn down their natural response.

When our cells become less responsive to insulin the condition is known as insulin resistance and it is a massive health problem today. With declining insulin sensitivity, our body tries to compensate by releasing even more insulin ('shouting even louder') and a terrible downward spiral begins. Eventually, our pancreas becomes exhausted and unable to produce sufficient amounts of insulin. This is diabetes. A disease where our blood sugar level stays high after each meal, causing oxidative stress, inflammation and glycation to become even worse.

After hearing all this, it may not come as a surprise that people who look young for their chronological age generally tend to have lower blood sugar and insulin levels. Similarly, centenarians are often found to benefit from low blood sugar and insulin levels; those people who produce less insulin over their lifetime have been shown to live longer.

For all of these reasons, you should try and keep your blood sugar and insulin levels down as much as possible. You can do this by avoiding foods that contain sugar and cutting down on foods that are broken down into sugar in your body. This is one of the most impactful things you can do to future proof your skin and, in fact, future proof your whole body and mind. You may think that by avoiding candy (sweets), chocolate, cakes and desserts, you are safe – far from it.

Hidden sugar

It is astonishing how much hidden sugar there is in food! These include canned vegetables, salad dressings, tomato ketchup, fruit yoghurts, soups and even supposedly 'healthy' snack bars. And don't just think about conventional table sugar in foods. Table sugar contains sucrose (saccharose), a disaccharide made up of one molecule of glucose and one molecule of fructose. So, if you see the word sugar, sucrose or saccharose on the label, there is no doubt that the food contains sugar. However, sugar may also be hiding on the label as corn syrup, barley malt, malt syrup, cane-juice crystals, caramel, dextran, fruit juice, fruit juice concentrate, molasses, maltodextrin, glucose, dextrose, polydextrose, fructose (fruit sugar), lactose (milk sugar), maltose (malt sugar) and many others. Any ingredient on the list ending with -ose should always make you suspicious but, as you see, there are numerous ways of 'hiding' sugar on the label.

A typical Western diet is incredibly insulinemic, i.e. it releases masses of insulin. This begins with breakfast, which is supposed to be a good start to the day. It is just the opposite! A typical breakfast, such as cereal or pancakes, is loaded with sugar and other refined carbohydrates. At this time of day, it is particularly important to avoid any 'sugar rush', as our natural cortisol level peaks in the morning and boosts insulin secretion after eating sugar-containing foods.

Natural sweeteners

Don't think that 'natural' sweeteners are necessarily any better! Many of them, including honey and maple syrup, make our blood sugar level shoot up just as much as pure table sugar and should also be avoided.

What about other, supposedly 'natural' sweeteners such as agave syrup? The much hyped agave syrup is very high in fructose, so let's take a closer look at fructose.

Fructose

Fructose is a common replacement for table sugar and is often sold to us as a healthier alternative. Agave syrup and many other 'natural' sweeteners have a very high fructose content (up to 80–90%). Another example of a sweetener extremely high in fructose is HFCS (high fructose corn syrup). It is present in countless processed foods and drinks, especially in the US.

I hate to be the bearer of yet more bad news, but fructose is no better than traditional table sugar (which is half fructose anyway) or glucose. In fact, in some ways, it is actually much worse than glucose. Just like glucose, fructose is also known to promote oxidative stress and bring about insulin resistance. And remember those Advanced Glycation End products (AGEs), cross-linking our collagen? Fructose has been shown to be even more active in generating AGEs than conventional sugar (Schalkwijk et al. Diabetes Metab Res Rev. 2004)! Fructose is also highly 'lipogenic' (i.e. it creates fat tissue), even more so than glucose.

Just one HFCS-containing fizzy drink per day has been shown to dramatically increase our risk of developing diabetes. And if this is not enough bad news, a recent study found that fructose promotes more aggressive cancer behavior and possibly even metastasis, i.e. spreading of cancer cells (Port et al. Curr Opin Endocrinol Diabetes Obes. 2012). In summary, you won't be surprised to hear that fructose-based sweeteners of any sort should be avoided like the plague. So, what are we supposed to sweeten our food and drinks with then?

Sweet tooth
First of all, it is important to retrain our taste buds to enjoy less sweet foods. We should really be aiming to cut out sugar and all sugar-containing foods, which will in turn also reduce our sugar cravings. Even zero-calorie, artificial sweeteners can elicit an (in-appropriate) insulin response and trick our brain into thinking that sugar was consumed (similar to a Pavlov's dog response). You might remember from biology lessons in school, that Pavlov's dog learned an association between being fed and a bell ringing, so the bell itself would trigger the dog to start salivating.

Retraining your taste buds to prefer less sweet foods is an important part of the Future Food Plan™. You will naturally lose your sweet tooth with time and that's a good thing. We are meant to eat a low sugar diet, it is what our genetic code is best suited to.

Such a change cannot happen overnight, it will take a little patience. It usually takes around three weeks to form a new habit. After retraining your taste buds you will appreciate the presence of natural sweetness once more and rediscover a heightened sensitivity to sweet food. For example, you might consider fruit to be astonishingly sweet, when you wouldn't have even thought of fruit being so sweet before. Trust me, I have been there and done that!

Sugar is also proven to be addictive (Thornley et al. Intern Med J. 2012). Therefore, the less you have it, the less you will crave it, I promise. However, to curb any persistent chocolate cravings, you could just have a couple of squares of 85% cocoa dark chocolate. I used to hate dark chocolate before I started the Future Food Plan™. I didn't even consider it as a food deserving to be branded as a 'treat'. However, with time my taste preferences changed completely and now 85% chocolate has become my ultimate treat. Alternatively, for some homemade chocolate recipes that are fully compatible with the Future Food Plan™, visit our website www.FutureProofYourSkin.com.

I am realistic in that we can't avoid sugar 100% of the time, but every little helps. For example, if I am invited to dinner and choose to eat the chicken with salad, there may still be sugar in the marinade or salad dressing. However, I have given it my best shot at that given time. And that's all you can do. So don't stress yourself!

Later, I will also tell you about an amazing trick you can use after having 'slipped' and eaten a sugar-loaded meal.

The good news is that there are some sugar alternatives available these days which aren't quite as bad. So, for those occasions when you really need to sweeten something, this is what I recommend. But don't forget about the retraining your taste buds advice!

Sugar alternatives

If occasional sweetening is needed, for example, when baking a birthday cake, you could use a mix of stevia glycosides with erythritol (for example sold as Truvia®). It does not elevate your blood sugar and insulin levels, but can have a mild menthol-like taste to it, described by the experts as a 'mouth-cooling effect'.

Alternatively, you could use xylitol, one of my prefered sugar substitutes. Xylitol is a birch wood extract with a very low glycemic index (more about that later). Yes, the person who came up with the name 'xylitol' should be sacked, as the highly 'chemical sounding' name fails to reflect that xylitol is not such a bad product and even comes with some benefits. For example, it is a known prebiotic (i.e. supports a healthy gut flora) and also has anti-inflammatory effects. When you compare the name 'xylitol' to 'agave syrup', the latter sounds all fluffy and lovely but, in my opinion, is much more damaging to our system. I would always recommend xylitol over agave syrup, but make sure you buy the natural birch wood form of xylitol, not the one made from genetically modified corn.

Fascinatingly, xylitol may even have some benefits for our skin. In a scientific study, xylitol was shown to increase the amount of newly synthesized collagen, increase skin thickness and protect against age-related collagen changes in the skin (Knuuttila et al. Life Sci. 2000; Mattila et al. Gerontology. 2005). Who would have guessed?

The downside of xylitol is that too much can have a laxative effect. In addition, xylitol does not dissolve in foods like sugar. If you need to use it in a smooth, non-grainy form, you should grind it to powdered form in a kitchen blender before use.

In the US, you can also get a chicory root-based sweetener (e.g. Just Like Sugar®), which has a glycemic index of zero and sounds like a decent sugar alternative. Like xylitol, it also has prebiotic properties, but unfortunately it is not yet available in the UK.

Artificial sweeteners
Just to make it absolutely clear – it is important to avoid any artificial sweeteners such as aspartame and cyclamate. They are highly chemically processed, unhealthy agents. Don't go near them!

The name of the game
So, what is the name of the game to keeping your skin look young? Yes – it is keeping blood sugar and insulin levels down to minimize inflammation, oxidative stress and glycation!

Oh, I haven't told you yet about the other revelation in my old diary, have I? When going through the entries, I was really shocked to read about a completely 'forgotten' health issue I had discovered at the time. My doctor had diagnosed a so-called 'pathological glucose tolerance' which, in plain English, means that I was borderline diabetic. Today, it is beyond me how I could have just ignored and subsequently forgotten about this important fact for nearly two decades. I guess in your twenties you feel invincible and, because diabetes didn't fit into my personal life plan, I buried the information in the deepest recesses of my brain. Goodness knows what damage I did to my body and skin in the intervening years by not adjusting my lifestyle. However, this is one more reason to stick to the Future Food Plan™ and keep future proofing myself – it's never too late to start to be good!

Remember ...
- Keep your blood sugar and insulin level down to reduce oxidative stress, glycation and inflammation
- Avoid all sugar and sugar-containing foods
- Avoid artificial sweeteners
- Avoid sweeteners high in fructose including natural sweeteners
- Avoid fructose-containing processed foods and drinks

Chapter 4

The grain of truth

In the last chapter, I shared lots of scientific evidence to show that consuming sugar is bad for us. Hopefully, I convinced you to avoid sugar and all sugar-containing foods from now on. If you are honest with yourself, I suspect you always knew that sugar was no good for you – am I right? But now comes the controversial part!

The vast majority of people today still believe that a diet rich in grains is good for our health. This belief is particularly common amongst people who are trying hard to live a healthy and 'clean' life. This advice is also a feature of the official 'healthy' eating food pyramid, which places the greatest emphasis on grain-based carbohydrates at the bottom and fat at the very tip of the pyramid. This needs serious rethinking!

The truth about grains
Let me tell you something you may not know. The carbohydrates in grains, i.e. starch, are simply long strings of sugar molecules! Starch is essentially a plant storage form of sugar. If you don't believe me, read on.

You may remember that glucose (the sugar molecule our body uses for fuel) is a 'monosaccharide', i.e. just a single unit of sugar ('simple' carbohydrate). Conventional table sugar, the type we may heap into our tea or coffee, is a 'disaccharide' made up of two connected units of sugar (glucose and fructose). Starch, on the other hand, is a bigger molecule – a 'polysaccharide' ('complex' carbohydrate) – consisting of a large number of sugar units joined together to form a long chain. These starch units are called amylose and amylopectin. If you look at their chemical structures below, even without a chemistry degree, you can clearly see that amylose is a linear string of lots of glucose molecules attached to each other. When looking at the chemical structure of amylopectin, you will find that it is simply a branched string of lots of glucose molecules. After eating starch, our body ultimately breaks these linear or branched sugar strings down into individual sugar units!

Figure 1: Chemical structures of sugar and starch

Glucose sugar:

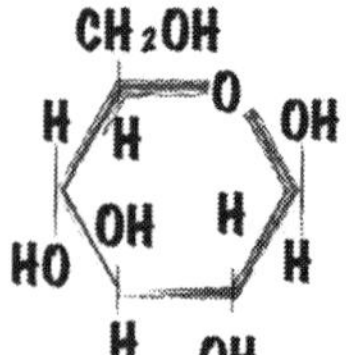

Amylose starch:

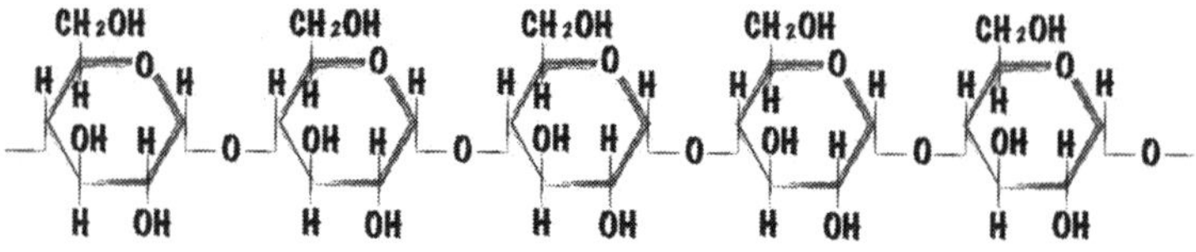

Amylopectin starch:

Carbohydrates are the predominant macronutrient in a Western diet. A common recommendation is to have at least half of our daily calories ('better' even 75%) come from carbohydrates and in many people this figure comes to 80% or even higher. We are led to believe that grain-based staples such as bread and pasta are particularly good for our health and that we should have lots and lots of them every day.

But when we eat these starchy foods, they are broken down into sugar molecules as described above. This digestive process starts in our mouth when we are chewing our food. Let's say we are eating bread. Our saliva contains an enzyme called amylase, and its job is to break down starch into sugar molecules. Try chewing bread for a bit longer than usual and you will find that it gradually starts to taste sweet!

This digestion process is completed in our intestines, where every starch molecule is ultimately broken down into sugar units. Eventually every 4g of starchy carbohydrates will result in one teaspoon of sugar in our blood. Did you realize this? So it is not only sugar, but also starchy foods such as grains, which elevate our blood sugar and insulin levels.

Most starches do this at a slower pace than sugar, but here's another shocker, some supposedly healthy, starchy foods can have a worse effect on our blood sugar level than pure table sugar! I will give you some examples later.

That's why a diet relying largely on carbohydrates is bad for our skin health and our longevity! It will make our skin and our entire body age prematurely.

When I see patients in clinic, we often talk about nutrition. I have lost count of the number of times patients reassure me that there is nothing I can tell them about healthy eating they don't already know. And I have no doubts that they are highly conscientious, trying their absolute best to eat healthily. They even tell me that they only buy organic produce. According to their belief system, which is of course fueled by the unfortunate current 'healthy' eating advice, they are really doing all the right things. However, on further questioning it often turns out that they are on a low-fat, high-grain diet. I am sorry, but a low-fat, grain-fueled diet is neither good for your skin, nor for your general health! I will talk about scientific studies confirming this in a little while, but first let's have a look at a commonly used system to judge carbohydrates.

What's wrong with the GI concept?

You may have heard that complex carbohydrates such as whole grains elevate your blood sugar and insulin level at a slower speed than sugar and refined flour. This is correct in principal. Let's look into the concept of how quickly a food elevates our blood sugar level a little further though. It is correct that different types of carbohydrates have different effects on our blood sugar level. Simple sugars such as glucose are absorbed quickly and cause a rapid elevation of blood sugar level after consumption, while complex carbohydrates such as whole grains lead to a slower rise.

You may have heard about the glycemic index (GI), a system quantifying how quickly a certain food will raise our blood sugar level after eating. GI ranks carbohydrates on a scale from 0 to 100. Foods with a high GI are more quickly digested and absorbed and cause a rapid rise in levels of both blood sugar and insulin. By contrast, low GI foods produce more gradual increases in glucose and insulin. The GI of glucose is arbitrarily set at 100 and all other food items are compared to glucose. Generally foods are divided into three GI groups – low (GI of 55 or less), medium (GI of 56 to 69) and high (GI of 70 and above). Closely related to this is another system called glycemic load (GL). This not only takes into consideration the general effect of a food item on our blood sugar level, but also the typical portion size of this particular food.

Countless scientific studies have shown that a diet high in GI or GL can cause chronic low-grade inflammation in the body and has numerous harmful long-term consequences. As persistent micro-inflammation accelerates skin aging, it seems a good idea to avoid any high GI/GL foods and go for whole meal flour instead of white, refined flour. In principal this is correct. A low GI/GL diet also has proven benefits for acne and other inflammatory skin conditions.

However, while the GI/GL indexes are a useful starting point when judging dietary carbohydrates, there is much more to the story as you will see later. But for now, let's talk just a little more about concrete GI values first. This reveals some truly surprising data!

There are many lists of GI/GL values, mostly published by reputable academic sources. When glancing over these lists, you generally notice that refined grains ('white' flour foods) tend to have a higher GI/GL value compared to their wholegrain ('brown') cousins. That's not a surprise and it's also true for rice. White rice, for example, has been quoted with a GI value of 89, while brown rice is listed as 50 (source: Harvard Medical School).

However, things are unfortunately not always that easy to judge. Let's have a look at bread for example: 'white wheat flour bread' is listed by Harvard Medical School with a GI of 71, while '100% whole grain bread' is listed with a lower (i.e. better) value of around 51, as expected. However, in the same Harvard Medical School food list, you can also find 'whole wheat bread' (which you would expect to be lower than 'white wheat flour bread') with a GI of on average 71. So the GI of this particular 'whole wheat bread' is as bad as the 'white wheat flour bread'! I am just telling you about this example to demonstrate that you can't blindly assume 'brown' foods have a lower GI than 'white' foods.

There are in fact many, many factors influencing the GI/GL index of foods including the type of preparation and processing, additional ingredients and a large variety of other factors.

For example, brown breads can be treated with enzymes to soften their crust, which makes the starch more accessible, leading to a higher GI/GL value.

There can also be significant discrepancies between different brands of the same food item. Sometimes foods are even presented in a misleading way deliberately – a bit of food dye goes a long way to make bread look browner and thus 'healthier'!

A bowl of sugar for breakfast
The thing that shocked me most, however, when looking at GI/GL indexes was that a substantial number of everyday foods, many of them supposedly 'healthy', have a higher GI value than pure table sugar! Would you believe that cornflakes and plain baguette can have a GI of up to 95 (source: Sydney University), compared to pure table sugar with a GI of 68? Many parents are giving their children cornflakes for breakfast on a daily basis. You may as well serve them a bowl of sugar.

Talking about children and trying to do the right thing, did you know that rice crackers (which I have given my own children in the past in good faith) have a staggering GI of 78 (source: Linus Pauling Institute, Oregon State University), again higher than table sugar! And steamed white rice is not much better. When I recently read about a supposedly super-healthy 'rice detox', where you eat nothing but rice for an entire week, I had to laugh out loud. That's one big, fat insulin bonanza (or 'Carbonanza'). Welcome premature aging!

Even foods considered as really 'healthy' options in mainstream opinion can sometimes have extremely high GI/GL values.

What about a baked potato with a GI of up to 98 (source: Sydney University) or 'oven-baked pretzels'? They sound like a healthy snack option. The 'oven-baked' implies low-fat and thus 'healthy' in our society but when they were measured, they had a GI of 83 (source: Harvard Medical School). Remember pure table sugar has a GI of 68. So next time you are going for a plain jacket potato for lunch with low-fat pretzels as dessert in order to be 'good', think again!

I think it is probably useful to summarize the GI/GL discussion. It certainly is a good idea to keep the GI/GL value of your daily food intake as low as possible and, if you have to choose between two different carbohydrate options, choose the one with the lower GI/GL index. However, don't forget that while blood sugar and insulin increases might happen more slowly with whole grain versions, you are still eating foods with a very high net content of carbohydrates. 'Net carbs' is what we call total carbohydrate content minus fiber. And all net carbs are ultimately broken down into sugar molecules in our body, as you now know. Also, the GI system has a blind spot for fructose!

One step ahead
So while the low GI/GL movement points us in the right direction, the Future Food Plan™ goes one step further. You simply can't assume that if we replace something that is bad for us (e.g. white flour) with something that is slightly less bad (whole meal flour), then lots and lots of that slightly-less-bad-food is suddenly good for us. No! If you are really committed to slowing down the aging process, hold on to your seats, as I will be proposing something quite outrageous!

I am in fact recommending that you do not merely cut out all sugary foods and stick to a low-GI/GL type diet but, for maximum benefit, you should greatly reduce or avoid grain-based foods entirely. This includes even those supposedly 'healthy' whole grains. This means no grain- or pseudo-grain-based foods including wheat, rye, barley, millet, oats, spelt, kamut, quinoa, buckwheat, rice, amaranth, sorghum, corn etc. Sweetcorn is not a vegetable by the way, but a corn (as the name implies) and should also be avoided.

This sounds radical, I know, and I will explain why it is important. But first, let me tell you why my recommendation is actually not that radical at all, but the way we are meant to eat and, in fact, have eaten for millions of years. It is in fact a perfectly balanced diet, much more so than what we are brain-washed to believe is 'balanced' eating. Bear with me!

Genetically we are still cavemen and cavewomen

Agriculture involving cultivation of grains was only introduced about 10,000 years ago, a tiny blip of time in the big scheme of things, given the Paleolithic era lasted 2.6 million years. If we compare human life from the start of the Stone Age to a 24-hour day, introduction of agriculture happened at around five to midnight. That's an extremely recent, massive change to our diet.

Before introduction of agriculture, we lived as hunter-gatherers and there were no cultivated grains. So, for hundreds of thousands of years, we lived happily on a diet with very low net carbohydrate content. Since the Neolithic Revolution around 10,000 years ago, however, the proportion of insulin-increasing foods such as sugar, grains (e.g. wheat and corn-based foods) and low-fat dairy products in our diet has increased dramatically compared to our Paleolithic ancestors. The excessive consumption of sugar and grain-based foods was further augmented by the Industrial Revolution some 200 years ago.

The human genome, however, has not had the chance to adapt to this recent switch in our diet and our genetic hard-wiring remains very similar to that of our hunter-gatherer ancestors, who were ingesting a far less insulinotropic diet. That's why our body is much better adapted to a low carb, high fat diet. The fact that our genetic make-up is not ideally suited to the current overconsumption of carbohydrates becomes obvious when you look at the soaring levels of obesity, diabetes, autoimmune diseases, cancer and heart disease. The prevalence of these diseases was unknown before the 'Carbonanza' era. The current mad 'Carbonanza' really is *not* a 'balanced' diet! With exploding obesity rates amongst children, experts are now even warning that our children's generation sadly is likely to have a lower life expectancy than our own.

You may interject that cavemen and women did not have a great life expectancy either. Well, it is correct that overall life expectancy has gradually been going up since the Stone Age but this is largely a result of industrial developments alongside the progress in medicine and public health measures such as antibiotics, surgery, vaccines etc. Our Stone Age ancestors did not have a shorter lifespan because of their diet, but for other reasons such as accidents, predators, infections, lack of medical support and advanced shelter. Anthropologists have also shown that a significant percentage of them died in violent, interpersonal conflicts. Most fascinatingly, however, life expectancy has not been rising consistently since the Stone Age. With the advent of grain agriculture it actually went down, before gradually moving upwards again! Did you also know that when man introduced grains into our diet, our body height and brain size decreased?

It is also interesting to note that while Paleolithic people had fairly healthy teeth with almost no caries, during Neolithic times, with its ample supply of carbohydrate-based foods, the rates of caries went up dramatically (Richards. EJCN. 2002). Richards also confirms that the gradual spread of agriculture throughout the Old and New Worlds was often associated with a decline in overall health and body stature. With all this evidence in mind, it is crucial to re-align our nutrition with our genetic profile and re-adopt some of the beneficial characteristics of a more pre-agricultural diet.

What does our body really need?

Let's start off some with some important principles. Fats are crucial structural components not only for our skin but for our entire body. For example, phospholipids and cholesterol are abundant in each cell membrane. Some fatty acids are even 'essential', meaning our body cannot produce them so they have to be provided via our diet. Amino acids, the base elements of proteins, also provide vital building blocks for the human body and are crucial for cellular maintenance. Some of the amino acids are also 'essential' and have to be ingested with our diet.

Certain sugar compounds are also used as structural components in our body. An example of this is hyaluronic acid in our skin. In addition, carbohydrates are used as 'fuel' (energy supply) for us. However, unlike fat and protein, dietary ingestion of carbohydrates is not required for survival as the human body can manufacture all that it needs.

But don't worry. Despite the fact that strictly speaking we don't need to eat carbohydrates at all to thrive, I am not suggesting that you omit them completely from your diet. In fact, some carbohydrate intake is actually beneficial for us. But, for now, let's just say that we will be moderating our intake of carbohydrates and cutting out those that are least advantageous.

'Fuel' for our systems

Most people with a typical Western diet rely on carbohydrates as their primary energy source. However, our body is perfectly capable of using alternative types of 'fuel' such as fat and ketones (I will come back to ketones later). There are only a few systems in our body, for example the brain and red blood cells, which prefer sugar as a source of energy (although the brain is also perfectly capable of utilizing ketones).

With the Future Food Plan™, you will be eating more than enough carbohydrates to keep any glucose-dependent systems going. However, your body also has several clever back-up mechanisms, which allow it to generate glucose internally, for example from protein. This process is called gluconeogenesis and it allows our body to generate glucose on an as-needed-basis. It performs this function like a finely tuned instrument, without the unnecessary flooding of our system with overwhelming blood sugar and insulin levels as so often happens in a typical Western diet.

From an evolutionary standpoint, we are not designed to run predominantly on sugar energy, as this was a luxury in our ancestors' times. So we really don't need those mountains of carbohydrates typical of a Western diet. They actually do more harm than good – remember glycation, oxidative stress and inflammation!

It's carbohydrates that make you fat

A diet too high in net carbohydrates elevates our blood sugar and insulin levels and causes chronic inflammation. It also leads to the release of cortisol, one of our stress hormones, and the generation of free radicals. All of these effects are aging us prematurely.

And if that's not enough, do you remember that fat cells need insulin to unlock them in order to allow glucose to enter and be stored as fat? Insulin will also inhibit the process of breaking down fat. Insulin loves to create fat and insulin is the free gift with any high carbohydrate diet! It is therefore best to moderate intake of carbohydrates. To live 'low grain' is particularly important once you are entering 'middle age', as our body's carbohydrate adaptation drops drastically as we age (Fossel et al. John Wiley & Sons Inc. 2011).

What does that mean?

Avoiding grains in practical terms means avoid eating conventional cakes, cookies, biscuits, bread, baguette, brioche, wraps, rolls, pasta, breakfast cereals, pasties, pancakes, crepes, crackers, croutons, gnocchi, semolina, oats, corn, millet, barley, rye, wheat, bulgur, rusk, bran, spelt and couscous. Avoiding grains also includes pseudo-grains such as amaranth, flaxseed, buckwheat, chia and quinoa, although I consider them marginally less problematic.

Cutting out grains does not mean though that you will never be able to have cake or cookies again. I will show you how to replace skin-unfriendly carbohydrates in your favorite recipes with more skin-friendly alternatives. Have a look at www.FutureProofYourSkin.com to get some of my favorite recipes, including skin-friendly flapjacks, chocolate cake, 'Nutella®', potato mash and French fries. These 'Stefanized' alternatives are delicious, but won't make you age prematurely!

I can now hear you shouting out, "But whole grains are healthy". I do understand that we as a society have been brainwashed into thinking this our entire life. I felt the same until recently, especially having grown up in Germany with its bread obsession. When growing up, two of my three main meals each day consisted of bread. I wouldn't be surprised if they tried to strip me of my German passport for my outrageous suggestions in this book (better not translate this into German). It is extremely difficult to let go of messages like "eat less fat - eat more grains", which are ever-present these days. I am confident, however, that by presenting you with the newest scientific evidence, I can convince you that we do not need grains in our diet and that we are much better off without them (Sisson. Ebury Publishing. 2012; Jaminet et al. Simon & Schuster. 2012). And clearing away another common objection – rest assured that when following my advice, you will still eat plenty of fiber, from skin-friendlier sources than grains! So there is no need to worry there either.

Nature's toxins

There are more reasons to avoid excessive grain consumption. If you are taking your health seriously, you will probably be concerned about the impact of environmental toxins. You may, for example, buy organic produce in order to minimize pesticide ingestion. And that's a good idea. However, what we often forget is that nature also produces toxins and they are often where we least expect them.

Plants make toxins to protect themselves. Mostly, they are designed to protect them from insects, fungi and bacteria. However, certain plants have evolved to contain toxins that are disadvantageous even for mammals (Jaminet et al. Simon & Schuster. 2012). Seeds are often the part defended most strongly by a plant. If a mammal eats a seed-containing fruit, it is best if the seed itself is not digested, but passed out in the stool to help spread the plant offspring. So, evolutionary-wise, we are encouraged to eat the fruit but not digest the seeds. Apple seeds, for example, contain the toxin cyanide but thankfully they go through our system without being digested.

Grains are actually the seeds of grasses. We culture and harvest these grass crops for their dry seeds which are then ground to make flour. As the grasses don't really want their seeds to be digested, they contain ingredients that are not great for our health. This is supposed to discourage us from eating them. I apologize for this simplistic description, but this is what evolution comes down to, put in very simple terms .

Wheat contains a lectin, wheat germ agglutinin (WGA), to protect itself from insects, fungi and bacteria. WGA can exhibit insulin-like effects and has also been shown to promote inflammation, clotting and autoimmune disease (Jaminet et al. Simon & Schuster. 2012). Wheat also contains a protein called gluten, which can cause extremely serious health problems in sensitive individuals, and I am not just talking about people with classic celiac disease. Unfortunately 90% of people who are gluten sensitive, don't even know about it (Davis. Rodale. 2011). If you want to read more about the health problems associated with grain consumption I recommend reading 'Wheat Belly' by Dr Williams Davis', a medical doctor who thoroughly demystifies the 'healthy whole grain' notion.

Grains also contain phytic acid (phytate), an anti-nutrient that impairs the resorption of minerals such as zinc, calcium, magnesium and iron. Good resorption of minerals is critical for good skin health.

Another interesting fact is (although this might not be relevant to you personally) that a study showed that people supplemented with a phytic acid inhibitor experienced a significant improvement of 'botox' effects (Koshy et al. J Drugs Dermatol. 2012).

I am not saying that you have to avoid everything containing these compounds; nuts, tomatoes and green leafy vegetables all contain some phytic acid and lectins. I am suggesting that you avoid foods with a high toxin content and low nutritional value, such as grains. Against common perception, grains actually offer very little nutritionally (Sisson. Ebury

Publishing. 2012). They are just full of starch and little else. Eggs, fish, meat, vegetables, tubers and fruits are much more nutrient-dense, and therefore preferable.

Figure 2: The traditional food pyramid – low-fat, high-carbohydrate nonsense!

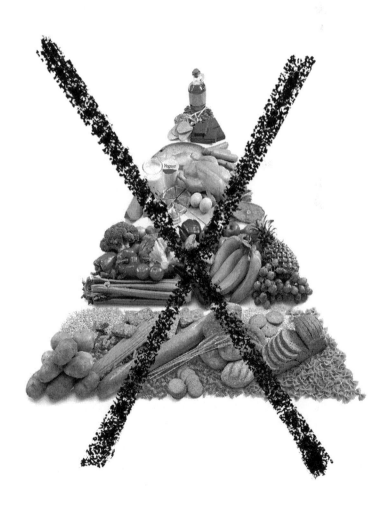

Why not go extremely 'low carb'?

After reading all this, you may be thinking why not cut out carbohydrates altogether and eat an Atkins or other very low carbohydrate style diet? Well, although carbohydrate overconsumption is disastrous, there are reasons why a moderate amount of 'good' carbohydrates may actually be most beneficial for long-term skin health and longevity.

The reason is that on a very low carbohydrate diet where less than 10% of energy is derived from carbohydrates, our body can develop a 'physiological insulin resistance' with time. This is a normal biological adaptation to a lack of dietary glucose.

As I mentioned before, our brain can use ketones for most of its energy requirements, but it also likes a bit of glucose. And keeping our brain happy is the highest priority for our body – our brain is the king! When our body detects that dietary glucose intake is very sparse, it does two things. Firstly, it produces more glucose via gluconeogenesis. Secondly, it will divert as much of the ingested glucose as possible to the brain. Cleverly, it does this by inducing a peripheral insulin resistance, preventing other tissues from guzzling too much 'precious' glucose. Remember, fat and muscle cells need insulin to unlock them to allow glucose to enter. Our brain is one of the few tissues that does not require insulin to facilitate glucose uptake. So, if our body makes our peripheral cells less insulin sensitive, glucose will stay in the blood circulation and there is more glucose for the brain to grab. Paradoxically, this means that the blood sugar level may remain higher than necessary after a meal.

For these reasons, not completely avoiding carbohydrates may have some advantages including keeping insulin sensitivity in optimal shape. I therefore advocate regular, but small portions of skin-healthy carbohydrates, in order to avoid development of physiological insulin resistance.

You have heard all the reasons why you should avoid sugars and grains, so to obtain your ideal portion of skin-friendly carbohydrates, I recommend eating a moderate portion of starchy tubers such as sweet potato, yam or winter squash (butternut squash). I prefer these to 'normal' white potatoes and rice, as they have a lower GI/GL value and a better nutritional profile.

This moderate amount of starchy tubers is in addition to plentiful vegetables and sensible amounts of fruit and nuts, all of which also contain carbohydrates. In general, the recommendation is to keep your carbohydrate intake to around 20% (anywhere between 10% and 30%) of daily energy intake and not the 50% to 75% that is typical of a Western diet.

It is important to eat your starchy tubers as part of a meal, and not on their own, in order to keep their GI/GL value as low as possible. It has been shown that eating carbohydrates together with fat, protein and fiber (e.g. fiber from vegetables) considerably lowers their GI/GL value. Also remember that the starchy portion on your plate should be moderate and never dominate your meal!

Other strategies for glycemic control include gentle meal preparation of your starchy tubers, such as boiling or steaming. For example, be aware that baking sweet potato in the oven rather than boiling it in water can double its GI/GL value! Industrially produced foods, processed at high temperatures, also tend to cause insulin levels to spike much more.

Last, but not least, adding some acid such as vinegar, can also improve glycemic control of starches. Vinegar has been shown in scientific studies to reduce the GI value and insulin response to a meal (Ostman et al. Eur J Clin Nutr. 2005).

I was an addict too

I have hopefully convinced you about the theoretical merits of cutting out bad carbohydrates such as sugar and grains. However, I understand that you may very likely be thinking, "I cannot live without them". I have lost count of how many times I have heard people declare there is no way they could live without bread and pasta! Trust me, you can. I understand that you may feel like this at the moment but this is because it is an addiction.

I see carbohydrate addiction as a true addiction, like nicotine. If you ask anybody to stop smoking, they will also tell you that they understand the theoretical harm of smoking, but that they simply cannot stop. A carbohydrate addiction is fueled by sugar rush, insulin release, sugar drop and subsequent craving for more carbohydrate-based foods. It's not a lack of willpower; it is a consequence of these simple physiological reactions.

There is good evidence in the scientific literature to support the existence of food addictions and there are many similarities between food and drug cravings (Pelchat et al. J Nutr. 2009). Two of the major players in our brain's reward circuit are dopamine and endogenous opiates. Cocaine, for example, is known to release dopamine in our brain and studies have demonstrated that the same can be said for food. Increased dopamine release in our brain may contribute to the development of addiction and therefore cravings and withdrawal symptoms when stopped.

Interestingly, the more comfort foods we eat, the fewer active dopamine receptors our brain shows with time, so we are driven to eat more to achieve the dopamine response we crave. It is a vicious circle. It is also interesting to note that the presence of opioid-like substances has been described in wheat (Schick et al. Clin Physiol Biochem. 1985).

But fear not, you can control this carbohydrate addiction! I have been following the Future Food Plan™ since 2011 and honestly, if I can do it, so can you! Seriously, I was the biggest 'carbivore' on the planet, literally living on carbohydrates such as bread, pasta, cakes and cookies. And the more I ate, the more I wanted (look at my 'before photo' on www.Future-ProofYourSkin.com and you will understand!). But once you stop, the cravings will gradually disappear.

Interestingly, if I now occasionally have a 'cheat day', for example when invited to a dinner or function and I am served food containing sugar and refined carbs, the addiction returns immediately. On those occasions, I find it really difficult to restrain myself and just have a small portion. But once I go back to the Future Food Plan™ at home, the cravings vanish. So, if a middle-aged, overweight, over-stressed carb addict with three jobs and three children was able to go cold turkey on sugar and grains, so can you! And the great thing is that you can still have treats and indulgences including cakes, simply in a skin healthier version. A guilt-free indulgence!

How to go for it

Notably, taking baby steps with lukewarm commitment to this revolutionary way of eating may actually be more difficult than going 'full Monty'. If you only half-heartedly cut down on sugar and grains, you are very likely to still crave carbohydrates and it will end up as a battle of wills. However, if you completely avoid sugar and grain based foods, you are much more likely to stop craving them.

Yes, you will have some initial withdrawal symptoms. These are only to be expected after all those years of messing up your metabolism. They may show up as a bad mood, slight lethargy, headaches or mild dizziness for example. The withdrawal can last (on and off, not constantly) for a few days or up to three weeks, but there are lots of tricks to help with the transition. During this time, your body gradually switches from being dependent on glucose as its primary fuel source to learning to utilize other energy sources such as fat.

When you start, make sure you have cleared out your cupboards of all bad carbohydrates and have plenty of Future Food Plan™ compliant foods available in order to avoid giving in and eating something 'forbidden'. I will share what these skin-friendly foods are with you over the next few chapters. During the period of adaptation, it is also good to have some nuts to hand, in case you start feeling a bit light-headed or feel like a snack, especially when out and about. In one of the later chapters I will talk more about nuts. Also have a look at the appendix for some Future Food Plan™ shopping essentials. The other thing to get used to is planning. I am always astonished how carb-heavy convenience stores and cafés are, containing row after row of sandwiches, cakes and the like. If you are lucky, there may be a salad lurking, but these tend to be dry, sad affairs and always contain some carbohydrate such as pasta. So you really need to plan ahead for lunch.

Also, when I go out with my family, say to relax in a café on the weekend, I often take a slice of my own Future Food Plan™ compliant cake along, so that I am not tempted by the sugar-loaded cakes and cookies on offer. Nobody has ever said anything, but you could always tell the waiter or waitress you suffer with food allergies if they disapprove of your homemade goods.

Also, be aware of emotional triggers for 'bad' eating. I know it's easier said than done, but being aware is the first step to minimizing the damage. To encourage a feeling of happiness within yourself and also to support rejuvenation from inside out (stress is shockingly aging – science proven!), I have worked with renowned hypnosis and brainwave experts to develop a groundbreaking 'Future Proof Your Skin' meditation CD. This is available on www.FutureProofYourSkin.com.

The withdrawal and adaptation period is over quickly enough and it is all worth it. Your body will successfully signal to your genes to up-regulate production of the proteins needed to efficiently burn other sources than glucose for primary energy. This is epigenetics at work – we are not mere 'slaves' to our genes, we can actually influence them! And there will be great satisfaction in knowing that you have achieved something amazing – for your skin, for your health and for your longevity. You have truly invested commitment into your future, a reason to be proud of yourself. Your body will have re-aligned with its genetic heritage and returned to how we are supposed to eat. It will have re-learned to use fat as its main energy source and, as fat is always present in plentiful amounts, you will benefit from amazingly steady energy levels throughout the entire day. Any feelings of hypoglycemia or lethargy in the afternoon will disappear as your body is no longer dependent on regular sugar fixes for its energy supply.

The good news is that after avoiding consumption of bad carbohydrates for about three weeks, you will have broken your addiction and will easily be able to live without them. You won't even miss them, as the addiction will simply disappear. The less you eat them, the less you need them. Then, the former, ravenous, eat-every-three-hours, sugar-burning you will have been replaced by an energy-all-the-time, fat-burning you.

For me personally, one of the trickiest things to adjust to was breakfast. I knew that a protein-rich breakfast (e.g. eggs or fish with steamed vegetables) would be ideal. However, I simply can't stomach eating something savory like that early in the morning. Most mornings I now have full-fat, live Greek yoghurt with berries and some nuts. Full-fat dairy is actually lower in sugar content and GI compared to skimmed, but more about that later. Other days I might have scrambled egg with blueberries or something similar. The blueberries make the scrambled eggs feel less savory, but make sure to add the blueberries at the very end otherwise they become all mushy and turn everything blue! Have a look at the appendix of this book to see a week's sample menu, which illustrates that you won't feel deprived in any way.

Skin friendlier alternatives

As I mentioned before, there are plenty of ways to make your new way of eating enjoyable and without having to feel deprived. The internet is an amazing source of ideas of how to recreate some of your favorite dishes without using skin-unfriendly carbohydrates such as sugar and grains. Try going to a web search engine and put in the name of your dish (say 'crisp'/'crumble'), plus 'recipe', plus 'paleo'. You will usually find lots of clever alternatives. 'Paleo' (derived from 'Paleolithic') or 'Primal' is the name of an increasingly popular hunter-gatherer type diet movement, which is in many ways similar to the Future Food Plan™, as it also advocates cutting out sugar and grains. So, if you are looking for new recipe ideas, 'Paleo' recipes are a good starting point. Just make sure you double-check the ingredient list, as sometimes they are trying to 'sneak' in ingredients which are not advocated here, but that's easy to detect. I found many of my initial ideas online and then adjusted them to my personal preferences and taste.

I can also recommend Maria Emmerich's innovative sugar- and grain-free recipe books, which contain delicious recipes for both savory and sweet dishes that are fully compliant with the Future Food Plan™. Maria also taught me that you can make a surprisingly good rice substitute using grated raw cauliflower, briefly fried in oil (not water). As a pasta replacement, she advises shredding zucchini into long strings and aubergine slices can replace lasagna pasta sheets. Instead of a bread crumb-based batter, you can simply use ground almonds with salt and spices (after rolling the chicken or fish in beaten egg). This comes very close to 'KFC chicken', but also works well with cod.

If you have a special occasion and want to bake a cake, there are great grain flour replacements, such as blanched almond flour and coconut flour. These flour alternatives for baking have slightly different characteristics, but you will find plenty of recipes online or check out Maria Emmerich's lovely cakes. Also have a look at www.FutureProofYourSkin.com for my very own black forest gateau recipe. It was actually a revelation for me what you can do without grains.

Although baking with these flour replacements creates lovely guilt-free treats for special occasions, it goes without saying of course that you should not base your entire diet on these baked goods, but have a varied diet containing lots of vegetables, eggs, meat, fish and healthy fats.

By the way, there is a difference between ground almonds and almond flour. For certain recipes, simple ground almonds (or 'almond meal') are fine and easy to get hold of (for example for skin-friendly 'KFC chicken'). However, if you want to bake with almond flour, make sure you get proper blanched almond flour. This is much finer and looks just like ordinary white wheat flour. In any case avoid any replacement flours made from corn, potatoes or rice.

Gluten-free?

So what's the deal with the explosion of supposedly healthy, gluten-free foods in our supermarket isles? Well, to eat 'gluten-free' is simply not enough. To avoid gluten but still indulge in other grain-based foods simply does not make any health sense, unless of course you have celiac disease, but even then you should take it a step further. Gluten-free bread is still made from grains and often actually has a higher GI than 'normal' bread. I have seen gluten-free breads with a higher GI than pure table sugar. So don't be fooled into thinking that 'gluten-free' is automatically 'healthy'.

What about legumes?

We have now established that we shouldn't eat sugar and grains, but what about legumes? Legumes belong to the Fabaceae plant family (Leguminosae). Grain legumes are cultivated agriculturally for their seeds (also called pulses) and include beans, peas and lentils. Legumes have a super-healthy reputation, but let's take a closer look.

Like grains, legumes have a high net carbohydrate content and also contain natural toxins such as phytic acid and lectins. Legumes also have an inferior nutritional value compared to animal products (fish, meat, eggs) and plants (vegetables, fruit). I don't have as much objection to legumes as I have to sugar (number one enemy) and grains (closely following as number two enemy), however, we can meet our carbohydrate needs with safer and more nutritious foods. So if you are really committed to long-lasting skin health and anti-aging, I challenge you to also avoid legumes, as I do.

In practice that means no beans, black-eyed peas, chickpeas, lentils etc. Peanuts and soybeans are also legumes and should be avoided. In fact, soybeans, although touted as healthy, are full of soybean lectins (soybean agglutinin or SBA) and one of the most artificially modified foods (along with corn) you can find. But because soy is a cheap source of protein, you can find it in countless processed foods, sometimes hiding as soy protein isolates, soy lecithin, soy oil or textured vegetable protein (TVP) among others.

Although also part of the legume family, I do eat green beans and sugar snap peas, as they are eaten with the pod and not just the seeds (it is the latter that contain the majority of pro-blematic elements).

In summary

To future proof your skin and body, remember to avoid not only sugar, but moderate intake of all grain-based foods and legumes. Remember that all carbohydrates we eat, whether they are 'simple' like glucose or 'complex' like whole grains, eventually end up as sugar molecules in your blood. And we all know that sugar causes pro-aging inflammation, glycation and oxidative stress, not to mention release of aging stress hormones.

Now that you know the things you shouldn't eat, let's get on to the truly exciting bits – all the lovely foods you can enjoy in abundance!

Remember...
- Grains and starches are long strings of sugar molecules
- Cut down on grains and legumes, as much as possible
- Avoid all processed and refined carbohydrates
- A moderate intake of starchy tubers (e.g. sweet potato, yam, winter squash, butternut squash) eaten with a fat- and protein-containing meal is fine

CHAPTER 5

Brain-washed into low-fat nonsense

Well done for listening to the list of things to avoid in the future. Now comes the fun bit! If we remove sugar, grains and legumes from our daily diet, what do we eat to make up our energy requirement and feed our body and mind? One of the crucial things is fat! Imagine – gone are all those miserable years of fretting about the fat content of your food and eating nothing but dull, dry low-fat stuff.

Eating fat won't make you fat
Before I go on to tell you why eating fat is important for skin health and longevity, first let me address a common fear – that this type of diet will cause weight gain. When I talk about the Future Food Plan™ and its high fat content, people become very anxious about the potential of gaining weight. Fear not, if you follow my advice it will not happen, in fact, the vast majority of you will actually lose weight. You will gradually gravitate towards your 'natural' weight, the weight that's best for your skin health and longevity.

I sometimes wonder whether anybody still thinks a low-fat diet is healthy or even helpful when trying to lose body weight. Interestingly, obesity rates actually rose dramatically in the 1980s, just after low-fat eating became very popular! This obsession was fueled by publication of official diet recommendations ('Dietary Goals for the United States') in 1977, which promoted reduced fat and increased carbohydrate consumption (La Berge. J Hist Med Allied Sci. 2008).

If you look at the graph below, which displays obesity rates in US adults over the years, you will be shocked to see that obesity rates only started to soar after introduction of these official low-fat diet recommendations. Since then, our society has also seen rising rates of diabetes, heart disease and cancer. I believe that fat has been unfairly blamed for today's health disaster, but I will leave you to draw your own conclusions when you have heard all the evidence.

Figure 3: Obesity rates (in %) amongst US adults aged 20-74 years (source: National Health and Nutrition Examination Survey NHANES 2012)

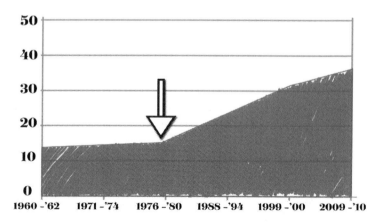

One thing I will say, however, is that I think there is an awful lot of lobbying going on, for example by sugar and grain agriculture industry groups. It is, of course, in their interest to keep the status quo (or even better, increase our grain consumption) and maintain the low-fat nonsense. I expect we will see a lot more of this lobbying in the near future as word starts to spread. I strongly believe, however, that within a few decades our children will look back at the current low-fat era and wonder what on earth we were doing.

And did I mention that the original 'healthy' eating food pyramid, with its large base of grains, was actually created by the United States Department of Agriculture? I don't think I need to say any more.

We really should not be afraid of eating fat as part of the Future Food Plan™. It is the bad carbohydrates that make us fat (and age our skin!). Eating fat will only significantly contribute to weight gain if we combine it with the wrong types of carbohydrates. Remember that we need insulin to unlock our fat cells? Well, we have much higher insulin levels if we eat a conventional high-carbohydrate, low-fat diet. Insulin also inhibits lipolysis (breaking down of fat) in our fat cells. The mantra is: carbohydrates control insulin and insulin controls fat storage!

And, of course, there are different types of dietary fat, some of which are highly beneficial, while others should be avoided, but more about that later. If you assume the latter are saturated fats, think again by the way!

Dietary fat keeps our skin young
So, forget the low-fat brainwashing of the past 30 years, our

body needs fat, and our skin needs fat! Let me tell you why. Lipids form a vital component of our cell walls (membranes) and help maintain cell structure and function. This is not only true for our skin cells, but every single cell in our body. However, clinical studies show that the healthy balance of fatty acids in our skin severely declines with age (Hayashi et al. Exp Dermatol. 2003).

A thought-provoking study confirmed that higher intakes of total fat, monounsaturated fat (such as olive oil) and even saturated fat are significantly associated with increased skin elasticity and decreased wrinkling of the skin (Nagata et al. Br J Nutr. 2010). Can I just repeat this – eating fat intake makes our skin more elastic and less wrinkly! Therefore, consuming sufficient amounts of fat is absolutely crucial to maintaining healthy and beautiful skin as we age.

There is another reason to avoid falling into the low-fat trap. When the food industry creates a low-fat food product, the removed fat has to be replaced with something. In the vast majority of cases, carbohydrates are added. And usually it is highly processed carbohydrates. Most of those supposedly 'healthy', low-fat, 'fitness' products are stuffed with processed carbohydrates, which increase your level of insulin, glycation, oxidative stress and create long-lasting chronic inflammation, all of which have an adverse effect on skin health.

Healthy fats on the other hand support optimal body function and are our skin's best friend. Fat also helps us to feel full and satisfied after a meal in a way carbohydrates simply cannot. And best of all, fat has virtually no impact on blood sugar and insulin levels. On the contrary, fat can even slow down the release of sugar from carbohydrate foods and thus lower the GI of other foods.

However, the consumption of unhealthy and chemically altered fats has led to all fats being viewed as a villain. So let's talk about which types of fats are most beneficial and which should be avoided.

What are fats?
Fats are a subset of lipids. Chemically, they contain glycerol and fatty acids and, as mentioned before, they are crucial for our survival. We can divide fatty acids into saturated and unsaturated types, depending on the number of double bonds in their carbon chain. Fatty acids without double bonds are known as saturated and the most common examples in our diet are those found in butter and animal meat. Fatty acids that have double bonds on the other hand are known as unsaturated. These can be further divided into monounsaturated (i.e. one double bond) and polyunsaturated (i.e. multiple double bonds). Monounsaturated fats (MUFAs) are present for example in olive oil, avocados and macadamia nuts. We eat polyunsaturated fats (PUFAs) in the form of fatty fish, many vegetable oils and many, many processed foods.

Let's start by looking at a very skin-friendly form of fat, the monounsaturated fats.

MUFAs
Monounsaturated fats such as oleic acid and palmitoleic acid have been shown in countless studies to have various beneficial effects on our health.

Different types of dietary fat:

MUFAs (monounsaturated fatty acids): These fats include oleic acid and palmitoleic acid. They contain one double bond in the carbon chain and are found for example in olive oil, avocados and macadamia nuts.

PUFAs (polyunsaturated fatty acids): These fats contain multiple double bonds and include omega-3 (e.g. in fatty fish) and omega-6 (e.g. in many 'vegetable' seed oils) fatty acids.

Saturated fats: These fats contain no carbon double bonds. A typical example is butter, but they are also present in coconut oil.

Trans fats and hydrogenated fats: These fats are formed when liquid fats are converted into solid fats by the addition of hydrogen atoms.

Avocado oil consists of around 71% monounsaturated fatty acids and consumption is associated with improved nutrient intake, reduced risk of metabolic syndrome and more healthy aging (Dreher et al. Crit Rev Food Sci Nutr. 2013; Fulgoni et al. Nutr J. 2013).

Olive oil is high in oleic acid, a monounsaturated omega-9 fatty acid, and been shown to reduce oxidative DNA damage by an incredible 30% (Salvini et al. Br J Nutr. 2006). Olive oil MUFAs are also associated with a lower risk of severe sun-induced skin aging in both men and women (Latreille et al. PLoS One. 2012).

There have also been countless studies over the years to confirm the health benefits of olive oil's phenolic compounds, including its antioxidant and anti-inflammatory activities (Cicerale et al. Curr Opin Biotechnol. 2012). Oleocanthal is a natural phenolic compound found in extra-virgin olive oil and has been shown to possess potent anti-inflammatory action, described as being similar to that of the medicine ibuprofen (Lucas et al. Curr Pharm Des. 2011).

Other MUFA rich foods such as macadamia nuts have also been confirmed as highly beneficial, able to quell oxidative stress and reduce inflammatory reactions. This is, of course, great news for longevity, slowing down our biological clock and skin aging, so we should eat lots of foods containing MUFAs!

Personally, I like to use macadamia nut oil for cooking. Not only is it high in MUFAs, but also offers a high 'smoke point' (around 210°C or 410°F), which means that the oil remains stable at higher temperatures. This stability is important for cooking oils as heating beyond an oil's smoke point creates unhealthy compounds. Avocado oil is another MUFA-rich oil with a high smoke point, around 270°C (518°F). I order my macadamia nut and avocado oils over the internet (available on Amazon for example), as they can be tricky to find in the supermarket.

I love to use extra virgin olive oil in cold dishes or to add after cooking, for example in salads or to pour over cooked vegetables. Olive oil is often quoted with a smoke point of 160°C (230°F), but its exact smoke point depends on various factors, as the case with all oils. Unrefined, virgin olive oils tends to have a lower smoke point than more refined olive oils (not that this should make you choose the latter though!).

Look out for the words 'mechanically pressed' or 'unfiltered' on the label to make sure your oil is as unprocessed as possible and hasn't been heated up to high temperatures.

PUFAs

Omega-3 and -6 fatty acids are polyunsaturated fatty acids (PUFAs). They require careful scrutiny as they can be a bit of a double-edged sword. Omega-3s (high levels of which are found in fatty fish for example) and omega-6s (found in many vegetable oils) both belong in this group. Three omega-3 fatty acids are important in human physiology – alpha-linolenic acid (ALA), eicosapentaenoic acid (EPA) and docosahexaenoic acid (DHA). Key omega-6 fatty acids are linoleic acid (LA) and arachidonic acid (AA).

Both omega-3 and omega-6 PUFAs are considered 'essential', meaning our body cannot manufacture them and they have to be obtained from food. However, maintaining a healthy ratio of omega-6 to omega-3 fatty acids in our body is absolutely crucial for long-term health. In the past, omega-3 and omega-6 fatty acids were ingested in roughly equal amounts, so we had an ideal ratio of around 1:1 in our body. With modern Western diets and their agricultural techniques, omega-6 ingestion has sky rocketed, resulting in a ratio of omega-6/-3 of up to 15:1 or even higher. This unbalance promotes chronic inflammation and can also promote insulin resistance.

A further problem is that both polyunsaturated omega-3 and omega-6 fatty acids are quite unstable due to their chemical structure. They both have multiple carbon double bonds which react quickly with oxygen, a process called lipid peroxidation. This cascading process leads to the generation of toxic compounds, which cause havoc in our skin and body, affecting health and longevity. The instability of PUFAs leads them to become rancid much quicker than MUFAs and saturated fats.

Omega-6

Out of the PUFAs, the omega-6s are the most problematic in our diet, not only because we are grossly overeating them (compared to omega-3s), but also because of their potential biological effects. Omega-6 fatty acids are the precursors for many pro-inflammatory mediators (i.e. molecules promoting inflammation) including prostaglandins, leukotrienes and other active molecules (Kang et al. Subcell Biochem. 2008). In addition, they oxidize very easily and can cause premature aging.

There are, of course, many more aspects to this but broadly speaking, omega-6 fatty acids are pro-inflammatory, while omega-3 fatty acids are anti-inflammatory. And although not all omega-6 containing foods are automatically bad for us, we should try very hard to reduce our omega-6 intake in order to optimize our omega-6/-3 ratio.

A large proportion of the omega-6 fatty acids in our diet come from processed foods and polyunsaturated vegetable oils such as soy oil, corn oil, canola oil, safflower oil, sunflower oil and other seed oils. Polyunsaturated vegetable oils should be avoided completely as they not only have a poor omega-6/-3 ratio, but they are also heavily refined. On pre-packaged foods, you will often simply see the term 'vegetable oil' on the ingredient list. That is enough reason to walk away! This may all be quite surprising to hear, as I am sure may people think of vegetable oils as beneficial, especially when compared to the supposedly 'evil' saturated fats.

Unfortunately, the ill-advised doctrine of replacing saturated fats with vegetable oils (supposedly to improve cardiovascular health) has led to vast over-consumption of harmful polyunsaturated vegetable oils. Check the labels of pre-packaged foods on the supermarket shelf and you will be amazed to find 'vegetable oils' in nearly all of them. I am shocked to see this cheap ingredient listed even on premium and supposedly 'healthy' products. Even olives are usually drowning in polyunsaturated 'vegetable oil'. If they would have used (more expensive) olive oil, rest assured that they would have let you know.

You will also find 'vegetable oil' on virtually all ready-made salad dressings, which often also contain sugar. Instead of ready-made salad dressing, simply pour extra virgin olive oil and some vinegar (ideally not balsamic, as this contains quite a bit of sugar), plus salt, pepper and maybe herbs, on your salad. This is all you need for a truly delicious salad. If you suffer with anemia, squeeze some lemon juice over the salad, as the vitamin C maximizes absorption of iron from green leafy vegetables.

The predominant type of fat in animal meat is of course saturated fat. However, meat also contains PUFAs. Unfortunately its omega-6 content can be significantly increased in animals fed corn-based diets. Ruminants such as cows are not meant to live on grains and corns, they are supposed to digest plant-based foods like grass. Even nursing lambs are often supplemented with 'creep fed' grains these days to enhance their growth. Pigs in the wild are foraging omnivores (i.e. they consume both plants and animals). In a natural environment they eat everything including leaves, grasses, roots, fruits and flowers. In confinement, however, pigs are fed corn and soybean meal. So when choosing your meat, make sure you select grass-fed animals to optimize your omega-6/-3 ratio.

What we should aim for is a balanced, healthy omega-6/-3 ratio of 1:1 to 3:1. We can measure this with a simple blood test. I measured mine recently and was pleased to see it was well within that optimal range.

Omega-3
Omega-3 fatty acids, such as EPA and DHA, have been shown to be beneficial for our skin as they are anti-inflammatory. They support healthy skin and also immune function. In a recent study, omega-3 was shown to prevent sun-induced immunosuppression in our skin (Pilkington et al. Am J Clin Nutr. 2013).

Supplementation with omega-3 rich fish oil has also been shown to support long-term skin health by preventing sun-induced changes in our skin and improving collagen metabolism (McDaniel et al. Wound Repair Regen. 2011; Pilkington et al. Am J Clin Nutr. 2013).

The benefits of omega-3 fatty acids are not confined to our skin, they are also good for our health overall. Omega-3 fatty acids have been shown to have anti-inflammatory properties, reduce oxidative stress, improve platelet and immune function, reduce the risk of various cancers and be highly beneficial for cardiovascular health (Mozaffarian et al. J Am Coll Cardiol. 2011; Kim et al. BMC Cancer. 2009). It has also been reported that omega-3 fatty acids are beneficial for telomere length, the marker for true biological age (Fossel et al. John Wiley & Sons Inc. 2011). In one study, those individuals in the lowest omega-3 quartile (i.e. with lowest levels of DHA and EPA) experienced the fastest rate of telomere shortening, whereas those in the highest quartile experienced the slowest rate of telomere shortening (Farzaneh-Far et al. JAMA. 2010).

Of the different types of omega-3 fatty acids, DHA and EPA are most beneficial; alpha-linolenic acid (ALA, found in flaxseed for example) does not provide the same health benefits. It is not reliably converted into active EPA and DHA, especially as we get older.

By far the best source of omega-3 is oily, cold-water fish. If you are taking fish oil supplements, make sure they are high quality, always stored in the fridge and contain high doses of the omega-3s EPA and DHA (not just ALA and certainly no omega-6s). This risk of oxidization during storage (i.e. rancidity) is naturally greater with fish oil supplements (whether capsules or liquid) than with fresh or frozen fish. You can sometimes detect a nasty fishy taste in spoiled fish oil supplements.

With regards to PUFAs, you now know that we should dramatically reduce our omega-6 intake. But there is one group of fats that are even worse for us than omega-6s.

What is the worst type of fat?

The worst types of fats are the trans and hydrogenated or partially hydrogenated fats, as they cause inflammation and premature aging in our whole body. They are generated during the processing of polyunsaturated vegetable oils (for example to make them more solid at room temperature). They are commonly found in most convenience and processed food including baked goods, chips, crisps, cookies, frozen pizza, as well as in margarine.

Trans fats and hydrogenated or partially hydrogenated fats are tremendously harmful to our health and we should try to avoid them at all cost. But be aware – just because the ingredient label reads 'zero trans fats', it doesn't mean there aren't any. According to FDA regulations in the US, manufacturers are allowed to label a product as 'zero', if it contains less than 0.5 mg per serving. So, by keeping the recommended serving size small, it is possible to massage the data. If you see any type of 'hydrogenated oil', 'partially hydrogenated oil' or 'shortening' on the ingredient list, it is highly likely that there are trans fats present, even though the label may claim 'zero'. In the UK, there has been a great deal of public pressure to eliminate trans fats from foods. Although their use has been reduced, they have not yet been completely eliminated.

Let's now talk about something highly controversial – saturated fat. Is it the evil of all evils as we are led to believe?

Saturated fat

There is a real hysteria surrounding saturated fats and we are constantly bombarded with advice to shun them. But, in reality, saturated fats are not as bad as their reputation would have us believe. They actually offer many advantageous properties.

Saturated fatty acids are an integral part of our body and constitute at least 50% of our cell membranes. They help prevent oxidative damage to cells too, so they are an important part of cell biology, both in the skin and throughout the entire body. I have already mentioned the study that revealed that people eating greater amounts of saturated fat benefitted from a better skin elasticity and less wrinkling (Nagata et al. Br J Nutr. 2010).

There has also been some rethinking about saturated fat intake and heart disease and a meta-analysis, which is the mother of all studies, has concluded that "there is no significant evidence for concluding that dietary saturated fat is associated with an increased risk of cardiovascular disease" (Siri-Tarino et al. Am J Clin Nutr. 2010).

I think the vilification of saturated fats needs to be seriously re-considered and I am sure that, with time, the current poor advice will change.

Saturated fats have even been shown to protect against the development of alcoholic liver damage, while polyunsaturated vegetable oil on the other hand is known to exacerbate alcohol-induced liver problems and oxidative stress (Nanji et al. Alcohol Clin Exp Res. 1986; Patere et al. Indian J Pharm Sci. 2011). One of the great advantages of saturated fats is of course that they are much more stable and far less susceptible to oxi-dative damage compared to polyunsaturated fats.

So, how come saturated fats have come into disgrace so much? One of the reasons may simply be that most people eating a diet high in saturated fat also tend to consume unhealthy trans and hydrogenated fats and over-indulge in sugary foods and refined carbohydrates. Think deep-fried (in omega-6 rich vegetable oil!) French fries and breadcrumb-coated meat, sugary chocolate bars and cakes. People eating meals high in saturated fat may also tend to go for highly processed, pre-packaged food, not to mention sugar-filled soft drinks. A very interesting study looking at life span confirmed that the combination of sugar with saturated fat seems to be the real problematic factor rather than saturated fat itself (Liedo et al. Exp Gerontol. 2012).

It is also worth noting that not all saturated fats are equal. I am a big fan of coconut fat, for example, which contains more than 90% saturated fatty acids. I bet you were always told that saturated fat will raise your bad cholesterol level, right? But, in a study published in the American Journal of Clinical Nutrition, coconut oil has been confirmed to raise the level of *good*, protective HDL cholesterol (Voon et al. Am J Clin Nutr. 2011). The study also showed that coconut oil induced these beneficial changes to the same extent as our friend olive oil (Voon et al. Am J Clin Nutr. 2011).

The saturated fat in coconut mainly comes from the medium chain fatty acids (MCFAs) lauric acid and myristic acid (Amarasiri et al. Ceylon Med J. 2006). MCFAs have been shown to improve insulin sensitivity and prevent metabolic syndrome (Nagao et al. Pharmacol Res. 2010). These coconut fatty acids can also provide instant energy, as they are easily digested. Best of all, they have been shown to reduce fat deposition and increase metabolic rate through heat generation (Noguchi et al. J Nutr Sci Vitaminol (Tokyo). 2002).

Butter is also rich in saturated fat and long been the arch-enemy according to most healthcare professionals. However, it is another example of a fat not being as bad as its reputation. Should you eat nothing but butter the whole day long? Of course not, but it is certainly better than eating the hydrogenated fat contained in margarine. Also, when cooking, saturated fats such as animal fats are very useful, as they have a higher smoke point than polyunsaturated vegetable oils.

Saturated fats in dairy products other than butter have also been vilified as harmful. How many of us have replaced cream and full-fat milk with half-fat or skimmed milk? However, recent studies have found that a higher intake of dairy saturated fat is actually associated with *lower* cardiovascular risk (Jacobs et al. Am J Clin Nutr. 2012).

A lot of today's health problems actually only started after people were cojoled into replacing saturated animal fat with polyunsatured seed oils. Omega-6 rich, unstable, polyunsatured vegetable oils are much more of a problem!

Sugar consumption has now finally been connected to a much greater risk of cardiovascular disease than saturated fat (Thornley et al. Intern Med J. 2012). I hope this is the start of more research evaluating saturated fats, as I believe it is time to rethink our attitude towards them.

But, of course, everything has to be eaten in balance. I am not saying that we should gorge on nothing saturated fats the entire day. What I am saying is: don't stress about saturated fats.

Cholesterol

And at the same time, don't stress about eating cholesterol-rich foods either! We have been advised to minimize cholesterol consumption for decades now, in the hope of lowering our blood cholesterol level. However, only a small part of our body's cholesterol content actually comes from food ('dietary cholesterol'). Our body synthesizes the majority of its cholesterol itself and that is for a reason. Cholesterol is an important component in our physiology. For example, it is the precursor of sex hormones and vitamin D, and an integral part of our skin. Like saturated fat, cholesterol has also been shown to protect against alcoholic liver damage (Nanji et al. Alcohol Clin Exp Res. 1986).

While dietary cholesterol has been vilified over decades, we now see more and more studies being published that doubt its harmful effects. This includes the 'evil' egg. For many, many years, eggs have been positioned as `bad' because they are cholesterol rich. I remember having discussions with my parents about not being allowed a second egg for Sunday breakfast as a child, because one egg per week was supposedly more than enough. I am glad to see new studies revealing that eggs are, in fact, a very healthy food (Kanter et al. Adv Nutr. 2012; Blesso et al. Food Funct. 2013; Blesso et al. Metabolism. 2013; Fernandez Curr Opin Clin Nutr Metab Care. 2012).

Blood investigations

Despite all this, it does no harm to keep an eye on your blood lipid profile by asking your doctor to take a little blood sample occasionally (after fasting for 12 hours). You need to make sure that he does not just measure your 'total cholesterol' (which doesn't tell us anything), but also asks the laboratory to determine both the 'good' (HDL – high density lipoprotein) and the 'bad' (LDL – low density lipoprotein) cholesterol. HDL helps in clearing away LDL particles, so you want to have a high level of HDL.

Newest research shows that not even all LDL is bad. Only a subgroup of LDL (small, dense LDL) is the culprit, the other subtype (bigger, fluffy, low-density LDL) is fine. Small, dense LDL has a much higher risk of being oxidized and oxidized LDL is the real problem. The LDL subtypes can easily be measured in the blood but it is not routinely done, so you may have to specifically ask for the test. I am happy to report that my HDL is in excellent shape and I have *no* detectable small, dense LDL, despite eating lots of saturated fat and cholesterol containing foods. I am only telling you this to reassure you and counter the near hysterical fear associated with eating saturated fat and cholesterol.

In addition to cholesterol subtypes, it is also wise to have your triglyceride (another type of blood lipids) levels measured occasionally to make sure they stay within healthy limits. Triglycerides can be connected to cardiovascular diseases including heart attacks and strokes (Austin et al. Am J Cardiol. 1998; Sarwar et al. Circulation. 2007). The interesting point, though, is that it is not saturated fats that make your triglyceride and small, dense LDL levels soar, but carbohydrates (Haffner et al. JAMA. 1990, Davis. Rodale. 2011)! A systematic review of the literature confirmed that a low-carbohydrate type diet reduces cardiovascular risk factors including triglyceride levels (Santos et al. Obes Rev. 2012).

Another useful ratio to be aware of in your blood is that of triglycerides to HDL cholesterol (Tri/HDL ratio). The lower your triglyceride level and/or the higher your HDL level (i.e. the smaller the ratio) then the better your health. A high ratio has been shown to predict heart disease (Da Luz et al. Clinics. 2008). This Tri/HDL ratio can also indirectly predict the LDL particle size.

Remember ...

- Your body and your skin need (healthy) fats; forget low-fat diets!
- Monounsaturated fats (e.g. olive oil, avocado oil, macadamia nut oil) and medium-chain saturated fats (e.g. coconut oil) are particularly good
- Saturated animal fats are also fine
- Full-fat dairy is preferable to low-fat diary
- Do not consume any trans fats and hydrogenated or partially hydrogenated fats (e.g. in convenience and processed food including baked goods, chips, crisps, cookies, frozen pizza, etc.)
- Eat plenty of fish to increase your omega-3 intake
- Strictly avoid all polyunsaturated vegetable oils, high in omega-6 fatty acids (e.g. 'vegetable oil', soy oil, corn oil, canola oil, safflower oil, sunflower oil)
- Avoid all pre-packaged food containing 'vegetable oil'
- When choosing meat, go for grass-fed animals

In summary: eat plenty of healthy fats, but avoid omega-6 rich polyunsaturated fats, to keep your skin fit and well for a long and healthy life.

CHAPTER 6

Which comes first – the chicken or the egg?

We now know that, for optimal skin health and longevity, we should moderate our carbohydrate intake but enjoy plenty of good fats. But what about the third macronutrient group – protein?

As mentioned before, protein provides important building blocks for our body and forms muscle, hair, skin and connective tissue. Proteins are made up of smaller units called peptides, and these in turn are made up of individual amino acids. As some of these amino acids, are 'essential', (i.e. our body is not able to manufacture them by itself), we need to make sure we ingest complete protein with our food.

However, unlike fat, our body has little capacity to store protein. So when we stop eating protein, within a day or so our body will start to break down muscle and other protein sources for its amino acid needs. This also happens on a calorie-restricted weight loss diet. We often end up sacrificing precious muscle tissue in pursuit of fat loss.

To supply our body with all it needs, we have to provide it with sufficient amounts of protein on a daily basis. Protein consumption has also been shown to increase the release of human growth hormone (HGH, one of our 'youth hormones') in a natural way.

Generally, animal protein such as meat, fish and eggs, contains all the amino acids we need to support the biological functions of the human body in appropriate proportions. They are, therefore, described as 'complete'. Plants sources of protein (legumes, grains, vegetables etc.) on the other hand, even those touted for being particularly protein rich, such as beans and lentils, contain considerably less protein than animal sources. Apart from very few exceptions, plant protein is also often missing one or more of the full range of amino acids. I therefore recommend eating not only plants, but also animal based foods to obtain your daily protein quota.

How much protein do we need?
However, while it's crucial to eat sufficient amounts of complete proteins each day, we should avoid eating disproportionate amounts when trying to optimize longevity. Firstly, excess protein can be converted into sugar by our body (gluconeogenesis). Secondly, studies show that while a very high protein intake may be useful for people primarily wanting to build muscle or lose weight, it may have adverse effects on longevity (Dussutour et al. Proc Biol Sci. 2012; Fanson et al. Age (Dordr). 2012). Most of these studies have been carried out in fruit flies or other insects, as life span studies in mammals (let alone humans) are understandably tricky. Therefore, we can't automatically presume this applies to humans but it is a good indication.

In summary, it is best to aim for an adequate, but not excessive intake of protein (preferably animal) each day. But how much is adequate? There are complicated ways of calculating our ideal daily protein intake, which take into account our body's percentage of muscle versus fat, our activity level, gender, age and many other factors. However, this is not a realistic method to follow on a daily basis. Instead of being hung up on exact protein intake, it is best to let common sense prevail. But, we can do some easy calculations to point us in the right direction. The current official recommendation for daily protein intake is 0.8g per kg bodyweight (which is equivalent to 0.36g protein per pound of bodyweight). However, protein requirements can go up to 1.8g or even 2g per kg bodyweight in very active people as our muscles need more protein when exercising.

For most people, our protein requirements would be 40-80g of pure protein each day, depending on body weight, lifestyle etc. Different food items contain varying proportions of protein depending on the amount of water, fat etc. present. On average, one ounce (approximately 30g) of meat or fish contains around 7g of pure protein. So a typical chicken breast for example, may contain 30g of pure protein, a fish fillet about 22g, a pork chop 22g, a steak 42g and one large egg may contain 6g of pure protein.

These quick calculations show us that it is rather difficult to overeat on protein if we let common sense prevail. Paul and Shou-Ching Jaminet recommend we eat up to around one pound (16 ounces or around 0.45kg) of animal foods (meat, fish and eggs) per day (Jaminet et al. Simon & Schuster. 2012), which I think sounds reasonable. The important thing is not to neglect our plant intake by over-eating meat, but more about that later.

In summary, this is not a high protein diet. If you want to put a name to it, I would call the Future Food Plan™ a moderate-protein, high-(good)-fat, carbohydrate-reduced, very-high-vegetable way of eating, but there is much more to it, as you will see.

Fish
Fish is a good complete protein source. It is also rich in omega-3 fatty acids and other beneficial ingredients, providing anti-inflammatory and anti-aging skin effects. Fish consumption has also been linked to a reduced incidence of heart disease and cancers such as breast cancer. In a study by Fortes and coworkers, it was shown that regular consumption of fish is also protective against the most dangerous form of skin cancer, melanoma (Fortes et al. Int J Epidemiol. 2008). Fish is also very 'telomere friendly'.

So for best skin health and longevity effects, try to have fish at least twice per week (but forget about the bread crumb crust!).

I understand that there are concerns about toxin levels in fish (mercury for example), but, in my opinion, the benefits outweigh the risks, especially if you follow a few simple rules. In general, the bigger the fish (i.e. the higher in the food chain) the higher the toxin levels seem to be. Therefore, avoid larger fish such as tuna, shark and swordfish. Low mercury and very skin-friendly fish include Alaskan salmon, anchovies, cod, haddock, mackerel, sardines and freshwater trout. Pacific halibut is also a great choice. For a Nicoise salad, try using anchovies instead of tuna. Prawn, shrimp and shellfish are also a good protein source and fine to eat, although they tend to be higher in omega-6 fatty acids compared to the ones listed above.

Lastly, try to find wild, fresh-water fish as farmed fish is reared in sewage-like conditions and fed artificial food including genetically modified soybean meal (Bakke-McKellep et al. J Fish Dis. 2007). That's why farmed fish tends to contain higher toxin levels and also higher levels of omega-6 fatty acids.

Meat

Animal meat is a great source of complete protein and beneficial for long-term skin health. Eating meat is also in keeping with our hunter-gatherer heritage. You can have pork, beef, chicken, turkey, goat, lamb and game meats, such as deer, bison, buffalo, rabbit, ostrich, duck, quail and venison. Organ meat, such as lamb's liver is also ideal as, compared to the muscle meat we usually eat, it is more densely packed and contains just about every nutrient, including high doses of vitamins, minerals and essential fatty acids. I sometimes make lamb's liver pate at home, as a dip for raw vegetables. It's really quite straightforward to make.

The great news is that even fatty meat is allowed in the Future Food Plan™ as long as you don't overdo it. It is always important to maintain a good balance. Overall, it is best to choose grass-fed, pasture-raised animals, as they have the best omega-6/-3 ratio. It is also best to try to buy high quality, organic meat whenever possible, as non-organic produce can contain traces of hormones, pesticides and antibiotics.

One important thing to remember is to avoid nitrate/nitrite-treated cured and processed meats, such as ham, bacon, hot-dogs, sausages, bacon and salami. They contain a carcinogenic substance called nitrosamine and have been linked to cancer

(Liu et al. Nutr Rev. 2008). Processed meat intake even shows an inverse association with telomere length (Nettleton et al. Am J Clin Nutr. 2008).

You may have heard warnings not only about processed red meat, but also about fresh red meat and a possible connection to cancer and heart disease. I feel that the jury's final verdict on fresh red meat is still out, as many of the studies leave a significant number of questions unanswered. There are also a variety of confounding factors to consider. Red meat consumption has, for example, been shown to correlate with several lifestyle risk factors for cancer such as smoking, high alcohol intake, low physical activity, higher BMI and lack of fresh vegetable intake. Furthermore, it has to be considered how the red meat was prepared (frying at high temperatures, for example, can create harmful by-products).

However, while we wait for more conclusive data, I suggest limiting red meat consumption, especially beef, to twice per week for peace of mind and remember to avoid any processed red meat. It is reassuring, however, that fresh vegetable consumption can be protective against gastrointestinal cancers (Liu et al. Nutr Rev. 2008) and we will be eating lots of veggies in the Future Food Plan™.

Vegetarians and Vegans
As you read these recommendations on fish and meat consumption, I am sure some of you are thinking – where does that leave vegetarians and vegans? To be honest, it is much tougher to lead a truly skin-healthy, anti-aging diet without eating any meat and fish (especially if eggs are also off the menu).

If you are vegetarian or vegan for ethical or philosophical reasons, I applaud your high standards, but there is unfortunately a health trade off. If you have chosen this lifestyle for health reasons, please reconsider! It is not what our bodies are designed to do. Apart from the difficulty of maintaining adequate protein intake, while keeping your grain and carbohydrate intake low, you will also run the risk of several micronutrient deficiencies, unless you are using regular supplements.

Eggs
Eggs are another great source of complete protein. Forget the recommendations to eat only the egg white, propagated by the ill-advised low-fat brigade. Eat the whole thing!

Egg intake, in particular the yolk, has been shown to improve our levels of carotenoids such as lutein, lycopene and zeaxanthin and to increase 'good' cholesterol in most recent studies (Blesso et al. Food Funct. 2013). These carotenoids are known to be beneficial for skin health and often an appreciated ingredient in anti-aging supplements (Anunciato et al. J Cosmet Dermatol. 2012).

Contrary to popular belief regarding cholesterol, whole egg consumption can actually improve blood lipid profiles as well as insulin sensitivity, even to a greater extent than yolk-free egg substitutes (Blesso et al. Metabolism. 2013). Egg consumption is considered particularly beneficial on a carbohydrate-reduced diet (Blesso et al. Metabolism. 2013).

As a conventional egg yolk contains more omega-6 than omega-3, I recommend buying eggs with greater omega-3 content. The best approach is to obtain eggs from pasture-raised chickens (not to be confused with 'pasteurized'), as this results in a better omega-6/-3 ratio and also a higher content of vitamin E, B, A and D.

'Pasture-raised' is not the same as 'free-range'. 'Pasture-raised' means that the hens are free to roam outdoors and eat an omnivorous diet including green plants, seeds, worms and insects. 'Free range' chickens are fed the same corn and soy feeds as regular chickens. 'Organic' labeling does not guarantee pasture-raised either.

Unfortunately, the label 'pasture-raised' is not well regulated, so it pays to do your research and maybe purchase your eggs at farmer's markets or directly from your local farmer, where you can ask about the hen's living conditions. 'Omega-3 enriched' eggs from the supermarket are second choice, but pasture-raised is best.

Eggs from other sources than chicken, such as ducks, emu and quail are of course also fine and add variety.

Nuts
What about eating nuts? Yes, you are allowed nuts (other than peanuts) in the Future Food Plan™. Nuts are rich in fat, protein and antioxidant polyphenols. They do contain some carbohydrates, but the amount of net carbs in them is low, so they generate a minimal insulin response (Dreher Nutr Rev. 2012; Vinson et al. Food Funct. 2012; Ros et al. Curr Atheroscler Rep. 2010). In fact they have even been shown to reduce the insulin response following a meal.

Nuts are also high in fiber, which is telomere friendly, and helps compensate for the absence of grains in our diet. The other thing I like about nuts is that they are great as snacks and, of course, extremely useful for grain-free baking, as I have mentioned before.

However, as with most things, it is important to eat them in moderation and not overdo it, as nuts may contain higher levels of omega-6 than omega-3 fatty acids (and the Future Food Plan™ focuses on reducing omega-6 intake). I wouldn't worry about the omega-6/-3 ratio of nuts too much though, as many types of nuts including almonds, hazelnuts, pecan and macadamia nuts overall contain more monounsaturated fatty acids (MUFAs) than polyunsaturated fats (PUFAs).

Eating nuts, even though they contain some omega-6s, is not comparable to consuming highly processed, unstable omega-6 rich vegetable oils. Also, nuts have a very good nutritional composition overall and contain many minerals and natural antioxidants to protect their content from oxidation.

My favorites are macadamia nuts, as they are particularly high in MUFAs (oleic and palmitoleic acids) and low in PUFAs. They are also rich in antioxidant polyphenol compounds, but low in anti-nutrients such as phytic acid. Furthermore, macadamia nuts are a good source of thiamine, copper and manganese as an added bonus.

Studies have confirmed that macadamia nuts reduce inflammation and oxidative stress as early as four weeks after integrating them into your diet (Garg et al. Lipids. 2007). I have mentioned already that macadamia nuts can also be used in oil form and that their oil offers a high smoke point. So they are a great choice for anti-aging, skin health and longevity purposes.

Almonds are also a healthy option. They are not only full of protein (one quarter cup of almonds contains about 8 grams of pure protein), but also high in MUFAs, fiber, B vitamins (important for skin, nails and hair), vitamin E, calcium, magnesium and zinc. Their fatty acid profile is not quite as good as that of macadamia nuts, but they are still highly beneficial for our health. In a fascinating study, almond ingestion has been shown to reduce glycation processes in the body (Cohen et al. Metabolism. 2011), which also means they help with anti-aging.

Needless to say that you shouldn't eat coated nuts or nuts roasted in vegetables oil. Also make sure that if you buy nut butter (other than peanut butter) that it does not contain any additives such as sugar or vegetable oil etc. Always check the label!

Go to our website www.FutureProofYourSkin.com for my very own recipe for 'Sticky sweet chili nuts' – they are truly amazing! I always serve them when we are entertaining at home and they have proven very popular indeed. I have never given out the recipe before, so you are very privileged!

Many seeds such as sunflower seeds have a slightly inferior nutritional profile to nuts, as they contain lower MUFA levels, higher PUFA levels and a worse omega-6/-3 ratio. Seeds also tend to contain higher levels of phytic acid than nuts. So go easy on seeds, although I don't advise to avoid them completely.

Dairy

Dairy or not to dairy is a difficult decision. I don't think our cavemen and women ancestors consumed much dairy as it would have been a little tricky to milk non-domesticated animals. The trouble with dairy is that it can significantly raise our insulin levels. Studies show that milk products elevate your insulin to levels even 3- to 6-fold higher than expected from their corresponding GIs (Ostman et al. Am J Clin Nutr. 2001). Combining refined carbohydrates with insulinemic dairy creates an even bigger problem.

In humans, drinking milk also elevates IGF-1 in our blood, which we are trying to avoid. Remember that *lower* levels of IGF-1 lead to increased cell repair and are associated with increased longevity. Higher milk intake has even been shown to lead to earlier onset of puberty and menstruation in young girls (Ramezani et al. PLoS One. 2013), possibly also connected to IGF-1. Some patients report an aggravation of their acne after consumption of dairy products, although not every acne patient seems to have this problem.

So, in an ideal world we would cut down our dairy intake as much as possible. However, certain types of dairy are worse than others. Milk, in particular, is very insulinemic and therefore I would certainly advise you to cut it from your diet. You don't need it anyway, as there are great alternatives, for example unsweetened almond or coconut milk. Don't substitute with rice milk (high GI) or soy milk (very artificial).

Fermented dairy products such as yoghurt, kefir, sour cream and buttermilk are not quite as bad as cow's milk. These are milk products that have been fermented with live lactic acid bacteria cultures such as Lactobacillus. Fermentation of dairy products consumes most of the milk sugars and reduces IGF-1 content. It also improves their digestibility and is beneficial for our gut microflora. Moderate intake of cheese, most of which are fermented, is also fine. I really like goat's feta cheese in my salads.

Studies have also shown that consumption of fermented dairy products over six months increases your good cholesterol HDL (Kiessling et al. Eur J Clin Nutr. 2002). In fact, lactobacteria are highly beneficial for our overall health as well as skin health. There are trillions of healthy bacteria such as Bifidobacterium and Lactobacillus living in our intestines. We have more bacteria in our gut than human cells in our entire body. It is very important to maintain a healthy balance of gut flora and support these 'friendly' bacteria with probiotics. Probiotics also support body weight control.

There is well-documented evidence to show that ingestion or topical application of 'friendly' bacteria promotes healthy immunity and reduces skin inflammation (Peguet-Navarro et al. Eur J Dermatol. 2008; Reid et al. Nat Rev Microbiol. 2011; Gueniche et al. Eur J Dermatol. 2010; Bouilly-Gauthier et al. Br J Dermatol. 2010; Krutmann. J Clin Plast Surg. 2012). Probiotics can also improve skin conditions such as eczema and some cases of rosacea. But not only that, probiotic treatment has been shown to reduce sun damage, have anti-aging and even life span increasing effects (Guéniche et al. Dermatoendocrinol. 2009; Kimoto-Nira et al. Br J Nutr. 2007; Matsumoto et al. PLoS One. 2011). Interestingly, a combination of omega-

3 fatty acids and probiotics seems to be particularly beneficial and has been shown to reduce pro-inflammatory cytokines and even improve depression (Gilbert et al. Br J Nutr. 2013).

Because probiotics are so significant, it is important not to rely solely on fermented dairy product as a source. I advocate taking an additional supplement daily, containing high counts of probiotics such as L. acidophilus, B. lactis, L. paracasei and L rhamnosus, as it is not really possible to get enough from yoghurt or other dairy with 'live cultures'. I currently take a probiotic supplement with a total 10 to 20 billion microorganisms (CFU = colony forming units) per day (1 or 2 capsules in the morning and evening, containing 5 billion microorganisms each). As with fish oil supplements, make sure that they are stored in the fridge. There are also foods you can eat to create a helpful environment for these healthy bacteria in the gut, these are called prebiotics. Prebiotic foods are for example leek, onions, garlic and as mentioned before, xylitol sweetener.

But let's come back to dairy products. If you decide to have fermented dairy, I recommend full fat rather than fat-reduced versions as they contain less milk sugar (lactose) and so tend to have a lower GI. Interestingly, going back to effects on acne, a study also confirmed that skimmed milk had the worst influence on acne (Adebamowo et al. JAAD 2008).

Dairy fat, which is a saturated fat, has long been criticized as harmful and fat-reduced versions are heavily advocated. However, newest studies confirm that a higher intake of dairy saturated fat seems to actually be associated with *lower* cardiovascular risk, as mentioned (Jacobs et al. Am J Clin Nutr. 2012). Other full fat, low-lactose dairy (e.g. butter, ghee and heavy cream) is also fine in moderation as it is naturally not very insulinemic.

In summary, my current stand on dairy is that it is fine if used in moderation and is not milk. Try to go for organic dairy from grass-fed cows, not only to avoid those added hormones and antibiotics but also because organic dairy contains a better omega-6/-3 ratio compared to conventional dairy (Ellis et al. J Dairy Sci. 2006).

With regards to maintaining calcium levels without drinking milk, you may be interested to know that dark green, leafy vegetables and broccoli (as well as eggs, nuts, coconut and almond flour) also contain decent amounts of calcium. However, I recommend asking your doctor to occasionally test your blood calcium level for peace of mind. If you become deficient, you can simply take a calcium supplement. I can report that my calcium level remains absolutely fine on the Future Food Plan™.

Remember ...

- Eat sufficient amounts of protein (fish, meat, eggs) on a daily basis
- Moderate amounts of nuts are very skin- and longevity-friendly, macadamia nuts for example are particularly good
- You may eat moderate amounts of fermented dairy products, if desired, but avoid dairy milk
- When eating dairy products, go for full-fat versions, not fat-reduced
- Consider taking a high quality probiotics supplement

Chapter 7

Skin booster food

To recap, for optimal skin health and longevity, it is important to moderate your carbohydrate intake, eat good amounts of protein every day and indulge in good fats. We have now covered our three macronutrient groups. However, I want to talk about one particular food group separately, as they are so important. It is time to talk about vegetables!

You won't be surprised to hear that consumption of vegetables has been shown in many studies to be associated with skin health and longevity. As they have such an enormous, positive influence on our skin, I recommend that two thirds of food on your plate comes from plant sources!

Vegetables will form the large base of our new healthy eating food pyramid. Instead of grain-based products like bread, pasta and rice at the pyramid base, there will be vegetables. So our motto will be – eat more green stuff and less white and beige stuff! I will talk about fruit in a little while.

So what evidence is there to prove that vegetables are good at future-proofing our skin and our life? Well, there are countless scientific studies published in the international literature to confirm this.

An interesting skin study by Nagata and coworkers confirmed that greater intake of green and yellow vegetables is associated with decreased skin wrinkling in the crow's feet area around the eyes (Nagata et al. Br J Nutr. 2010). This is highly fascinating. Crow's feet are classic 'mimic lines', i.e. they are caused by repeated movement of underlying facial muscles. So, if consumption of vegetables can influence these lines, they must have a very significant influence on collagen production, skin elasticity and overall skin biology.

In a study by Fortes and coworkers, it was confirmed that high consumption of vegetables including cruciferous (broccoli for example) and leafy vegetables was protective against the most dangerous form of skin cancer, melanoma (Fortes et al. Int J Epidemiol. 2008).

But it doesn't end in the skin. A diet rich in plant foods is also associated with a reduced incidence of many common forms of cancer as well as a reduced risk of heart disease and chronic diseases of aging (Heber. J Postgrad Med. 2004).

Most intriguingly, there are now several studies which clearly show that high vegetable consumption is associated with longer telomeres, i.e. lower biological age (Marcon et al. Mutagenesis. 2012; Fossel et al. 2011, Tiainen et al. Eur J Clin Nutr. 2012 ; Xu et al. Am J Clin Nutr. 2009). Broccoli, tomatoes, cabbage, kale and sea vegetables have all been named as particularly telomere friendly. Of course, everything that is telomere friendly should be our best friend!

I could go on and on quoting studies confirming the benefits of high vegetable consumption, but that would be boring. But let me pose a question: why do you think vegetables have such profound benefits on our skin, health and longevity?

One of the reasons is that vegetables are very high in nutrients, vitamins, minerals and antioxidants, making them highly anti-inflammatory (Anlasik et al. Br J Nutr. 2005). Vegetables are also rich in fiber, so there are no worries about not consuming enough fiber without eating grains! Actually, you may be surprised looking at concrete numbers. According to Harvard University, half a cup of broccoli contains 2.5g of total fiber and half a cup of Brussels sprouts 3.8g, while one slice of white bread contains only 0.6g and one slice of whole wheat bread a mere 1.5g of total fiber. So, if you fill up your plate with vegetables, there will not be a lack of fiber. And that's good, as fiber intake is positively correlated with longer telomeres (Fossel et al. John Wiley & Sons Inc. 2011) and longer telomeres generally equal longer life. Soluble fiber also helps blood sugar control.

And here comes one more bit of research to convince you. A recent study revealed that increased vegetable and fruit intake even benefits our skin coloration in a way that makes us look more attractive to other people! In this study, these dietary changes were confirmed to have a perceptible impact on skin coloration within a few weeks. Most amazingly, this had a greater impact than tanning. The researchers went on to suggest that these changes in skin coloration may even make us more sexually attractive (Whitehead et al. Evol Psychol. 2012). Well, if that's not motivating enough to make you eat more veggies ...

Which vegetables are most skin friendly?
So which vegetables should we eat for optimum benefit for skin health and longevity? In general, we should eat as large a variety and array of colors as possible. Great options are non-starchy, fibrous vegetables such as broccoli, cauliflower, lettuce, Brussels sprouts, spinach, peppers, mushrooms, onions, celery, asparagus, zucchini (courgette), egg plant (aubergine), leafy stuff such as rocket, lettuce, kale, cabbage and other greens. These are all high in fiber and have a low GI. With regards to green vegetables, the darker the green, the better.

Broccoli and kale are two of my favorites actually, as they are ultra-longevity foods and also full of anti-cancer ingredients (sulforaphane and indole-3-carbinol can be found in broccoli). Sea vegetables such as kombu, wakame, other seaweeds and algaes are also great.

Ideally, we should eat a mix of raw and cooked veggies. You may be surprised to hear that you can actually eat spinach, cauliflower, zucchini (courgette) and many others raw quite safely. They are great options to add to your salad in addition to the usual suspects. When cooking vegetables, try to use as gentle a method as possible. Vegetables can also be the basis of great replacements of less beneficial foods: think egg plant (aubergine) chips, kale crisps and cauliflower mash.

If you think vegetables won't fill you up, think again! The great thing about the Future Food Plan™ is that we are not worried about (good) fat. So, to increase the sense of satisfaction and fullness, you can always slather your vegetables in extra virgin olive oil or even some butter. Adding oil is also important for resorption of fat-soluble vitamins A, D, E and K. Also, adding some pine nuts or flaked almonds will greatly enhance many vegetables.

You can see that while restricting sugar and grains, you can still enjoy unlimited amounts of our most nutritious and natural form of carbohydrates – vegetables. Yes, pile them on, no need to restrict these skin-friendly fibrous vegetables, unlike on some very low-carbohydrate diets!

Which vegetables to avoid?
We should try and reduce intake of most starchy vegetables (root vegetables such as parsnips and turnips). Their net carbohydrate content is quite high and their GI can be higher than pure table sugar. Roast parsnip for example has a GI of 97 (Foster-Powell et al. Am J Clin Nutr. 2002) versus table sugar with a GI 68.

However, I don't have as much of an issue with root vegetables (in moderation!) as I have with refined sugar and grains, as long as they are eaten as part of a meal and in a portion-controlled way. Also, if you boil them they tend to have a lower GI than after dry roasting in the oven.

Interestingly cooked carrots, another root vegetable, have a quite high GI, but are very low in their raw state. So why not try raw carrot sticks with homemade liver pate dip? Beetroot, by the way, has a comparably high sugar content also and should be eaten in moderation only. Sweet corn is not a vegetable, but a corn (as the name implies) and should, of course, be avoided.

The other thing to avoid is canned vegetables, as they are not only less nutritious, but can even contain added sugar! Try to buy vegetables fresh or, if not possible, frozen. Most nutrients remain intact that way.

Fruit

You may have noticed that I talk more about the benefits of vegetables than fruit. In general, fresh fruit is healthy, as it is a rich source of vitamins, minerals, antioxidants and other phytochemicals as well as fiber. However, many fruits are quite high in sugar (fructose, fruit sugar). Modern fruit cultivation has also rendered our fruit much higher in sugar and lower in fiber compared to the wild fruit of our primal ancestors.

So, while fruit in moderation is fine and can be beneficial for our skin, if you eat the right type (see below), you should be careful not to over-indulge, especially with sweet tropical fruits as they are particularly high in sugar.

Eating lots of sweet fruit can also slow down weight loss by the way, as most fructose we eat is directly turned into fat (Volek et al. Beyond Obesity LLC. 2011). So, having nothing but fruit for breakfast is not a good idea either.

The data on exactly how much sugar is present in certain pieces of fruit naturally varies as not every apple is the same. That also explains the great variation of GI values quoted for different types of fruit.

But there are some great, very skin-friendly fruits. Berries of all types, including blueberries, strawberries, cranberries, raspberries and blackberries are great choices. They are high in antioxidants while not containing disastrous amounts of sugar. Blueberries have also been named as particularly telomere friendly. Most berries contain highly beneficial compounds such as anti-inflammatory anthocyanin (the compound behind the red and blue color of berries), anti-cancer pterostilbene (a compound related to anti-aging 'miracle' compound resveratrol) and the phenol antioxidant ellagic acid. Berries are also high in fiber, which is telomere friendly. Both fresh and frozen berries are fine to use.

Thinking about fruit other than berries (for example apples, pears, grapefruit and melon), I would say that these are fine in moderation also. However, don't over eat them. But you should certainly limit intake of high sugar fruit such as grapes, bananas and mangos.

Absolutely fine and highly beneficial for skin health and longevity are, of course, also cucumber, avocado and tomatoes - yes, they are fruit, not vegetables. Tomato contains lycopene, which has proven anti-aging benefits for our skin. That's why many anti-aging supplements contain lycopene as one of their main ingredients. Lycopene from food is surprisingly better absorbed from cooked tomatoes than raw tomatoes.

You may be surprised to hear that you should completely stay away from dried fruit such as raisins, dried apricots and dried mango etc., as they are extremely high in sugar. In some cases, their sugar content is comparable to sweets and candy!

Remember ...

- Vegetables are your skin's best friend!
- Try to make 2/3 of your plate plant-based
- Eat lots and lots of fibrous, non-starchy vegetables, but moderate your intake of starchy root vegetables
- Eat a mix of raw and cooked vegetables
- Add good oils to aid resorption of fat-soluble vitamins
- Enjoy moderate amounts of low-sugar fruit, especially all types of berries
- Minimize high sugar fruit such as bananas, grapes, mango and other sweet tropical fruits
- Avoid all dried fruit!

CHAPTER 8

Spice up your life

Herbs

Herbs and spices are a great addition to any skin health and longevity diet. Not only do spices greatly add flavor and variety to your food, but they also contain bioactive substances, which can have immense positive effects on your health and skin. Due to space limitations, I cannot talk about all the herbs beneficial to our skin, but let me share a few examples.

Rosmarinic acid is a natural phenol antioxidant found in many common herbs including rosemary, oregano, sage and thyme. It fights the aging free radicals and has anti-inflammatory and anti-cancer properties. A recent study from Baltimore confirmed that an oregano-cranberry extract can promote longevity (Zou et al. Age (Dordr). 2012).

I suggest adding these herbs to your meals generously, as desired. You could also get some fresh rosemary from the garden, pour hot water over it, let it sit for a few minutes and then enjoy a home-made anti-aging tea!

Curcumin, the compound that gives turmeric its yellow color, has anti-inflammatory properties and protects against cancer by inducing programmed death of cancer cells ('cell suicide' or 'apoptosis' of bad cells). Studies have shown that populations eating lots of curcumin also have significantly lower rates of dementia, a notorious disease of aging.

In a study done in human skin fibroblasts, curcumin was confirmed to stimulate cellular antioxidant defenses (Lima et al. Mol Nutr Food Res. 2011). Fibroblasts are one of the most important cell types in our skin as they produce our collagen and elastin.

Cinnamon is also beneficial. It is not only high in nutrients but has also been shown to help regulate blood sugar levels, reduce bad cholesterol and have anti-inflammatory and anti-cancer properties (Hong et al. BMC Complement Altern Med. 2012). And best of all, it can replace some of the sugar in sweet dishes. I always add cinnamon to my homemade FutureFood Plan™ crisp/crumble (go to www.FutureProofYourSkin.com to get my personal recipe).

Cloves have been described as 'cinnamon on steroids'. Of all spices, they seem to have one of the highest ORAC scores (Oxygen Radical Absorbance Capacity), meaning they rank highest in antioxidant activity.

Garlic has been shown to not only lower cholesterol levels, but also have anti-clotting, blood pressure lowering, blood circulation improving and cardiovascular disease preventing properties (Tapsell et al. Med J Aust. 2006; Rahman. Ageing Res Rev.

2003). Other claimed beneficial effects of garlic include anti-oxidative, antifungal, antibacterial and even anti-cancer activity (Svendsen et al. J Ethnopharmacol. 1994). The list is long, but I would specifically like to mention it has also been suggested that garlic can prevent diseases associated with brain aging and rejuvenate the skin (Rahman. Ageing Res Rev. 2003).

Garlic's anti-aging and rejuvenating effects have been confirmed in an interesting cell culture study, where the investigators looked at human skin fibroblasts and found that addition of garlic extracts greatly increased their maximum proliferative capacity (Svendsen et al. J Ethnopharmacol. 1994). This means these cells were able to divide and proliferate more often with the addition of garlic. The garlic extracts also improved other characteristics of skin cells in this study (Svendsen et al. J Ethnopharmacol. 1994). Garlic has also been described as particularly telomere friendly.

Other herbs and spices with reported benefits on skin health and anti-aging include basil (loaded with antioxidants that can protect your cells from harmful free radicals), marjoram (aids a good night's sleep, which is essential to cell regeneration), ginger (anti-inflammatory and an immune system booster), and Jamaican Allspice (from the Pimenta dioica plant, helps keep blood sugar under control and thus reduce the inflammatory effect of insulin).

Where possible, try to use organic herbs, as they have not been sprayed with pesticides. Herbs are plant leaves, which are dried and then left whole or crushed. As these leaves have a large surface area while growing and are consumed in their entirety (i.e. not peeled), organic origin is particularly important. I have developed an amazing recipe for oriental spicy nuts, which I also share on our website www.FutureProofYourSkin.com.

There is virtually no dish that fails to benefit from the addition of herbs and spices. Herbs and spices can also be used in recipes to replace less desirable ingredients such as sugar and salt, for example in marinades and dressings (Tapsell et al. Med J Aust. 2006). That brings me to the next topic – salt! Is salt really as bad as we are made to believe? Read on to find out what I have found.

Salt
Salt (sodium chloride) has important functions in the human body. We wouldn't be able to live without it. However, I acknowledge that most pre-packaged, processed foods are overloaded with sodium these days. Another reason to avoid pre-packed foods!

Apart from actual sodium intake however, what seems to be more important is the ratio of sodium to potassium (Jaminet. Simon & Schuster. 2012). A recent study confirmed that a higher sodium/potassium ratio is not only associated with a higher risk of cardiovascular disease, but even a higher risk of death overall (Yang et al. Arch Intern Med. 2011).

Interestingly, however, official dietary guidelines are failing us in this area. There is a peer-reviewed study suggesting that it is not actually possible to meet the official 2010 Dietary Guidelines for sodium and potassium simultaneously (Maillot et al. Nutr Res. 2013). The Guidelines have also been criticized regarding their recommendations for adults aged over 50 years; the official sodium goal of less than 1500 mg/day is actually not feasible (Maillot et al. Am J Prev Med. 2012).

The other thing to bear in mind is that the Future Food Plan™ will change your need for salt! The reason is that a typical high carbohydrate diet makes our kidneys retain salt, whereas a reduced carbohydrate intake increases sodium excretion by the kidneys (Volek et al. Beyond Obesity LLC. 2011).

For ideal health, try to increase potassium intake from plant sources (e.g. from green leafy vegetables, tomatoes, sweet potatoes and avocados), rather than worrying about slashing your sodium intake.

What about sea salt?

Sea salt and table salt actually contain quite similar amounts of sodium, despite the fact that sea salt is often marketed as a healthier alternative. However, sea salt is produced through evaporation of ocean water which, depending on the water source, may leave behind some trace minerals and elements. Table salt is usually more heavily processed and often contains additives, for example those to prevent clumping plus, in some cases, iodine and fluoride.

Professor Bruce Neal, Chair of Vascular Epidemiology and Prevention Medicine at the University of Sydney says that the only 'healthier' salts are salt substitutes which are lower in sodium chloride and higher in potassium chloride (plus a little magnesium chloride for taste).

I tend to use a special high potassium salt or pink 'Himalayan rock salt'. The latter is thought to be the least processed salt, contains some additional minerals and I simply like the taste. However, there are no substantiated health benefits for rock salt, as it still contains large amounts of sodium chloride.

In summary, instead of over-salting, use plenty of spices and herbs, but don't over-stress to please the anti-salt campaigners. Adding spices to your cooking won't just spice up your meal, it may even prolong your life. The good news is also that when you follow the Future Food Plan™, you will naturally be consuming less sodium anyway, as you won't be eating processed foods, plus your kidneys will excrete more.

Remember ...
- Use plenty of herbs and spices, as many of them offer skin- and longevity-friendly properties
- Increase potassium intake from plant sources (e.g. from green leafy vegetables, tomatoes, sweet potatoes and avocados), rather than forcing a low-sodium intake
- Avoid all (over-salted) processed foods

CHAPTER 9

What turns water into an anti-aging elixir?

I keep hearing patients in my clinic say, "My skin is really dry, although I drink lots of water". Unfortunately, the link isn't that straightforward. Skin hydration depends more on the lipids and water-holding molecules in our skin than the amount of water we drink. Having said that, we should of course drink sufficient amounts of water every day. But how much exactly is sufficient? Unfortunately I can't answer that question, as there are no scientific data to clarify.

I am sure you have heard it said countless times, "Drink eight glasses of water every day", but is that really true? Astonishingly, the eight-glass-rule does not have scientific backing (Valtin. Am J Physiol Regul Integr Comp Physiol. 2002). So while I certainly advocate drinking plenty of water throughout the day, there is no need to obsess about the exact amount.

It is important though that you drink the right type of water and reduce your intake of unnecessary harmful toxins. Water from plastic bottles for example may contain toxins, which can leach from the plastic into the water (Shotyk. Environ. Monit.

2006; Geens et al. Int J Hyg Environ Health. 2011). Glass containers are much better.

Unfortunately tap water is not necessarily any better than bottled water as contaminations can also be present. For example, nitrate in drinking water has been connected to bowel cancer (van Grinsven et al. Environ Health. 2010). When I see the color of the water coming out of some taps, I really wonder what else is in there!

For many years, chlorine has been used around the world to disinfect our tap water. And the good news is that it keeps our drinking water virtually free of harmful microorganisms. However, I feel that drinking water from the tap is a bit like eating your turkey from the supermarket with the plastic wrapping still on. Of course, both the turkey and tap water need to be protected during transport to avoid bacterial contamination (hence the chlorine) but before ingesting it, we want to remove as many additives as possible. We should therefore filter our tap water.

There are different types of filters, all of which remove different types of contamination. The most common ones are pitcher or jug style point-of-use filters. They reduce impurities such as chlorine, sediment, heavy metals and lime scale.

One problem with jug type filters, however, is the tendency to grow nasty bacteria over time. I have taken swabs from our office jug style water filter myself and found it to be contaminated with Pseudomonas! This can happen within a few months of usage so it's a good idea to replace your jug style filter every few months with a completely new one. Any slimy residue on the inside of the jug or its cover is a sure sign of contamination and a signal to throw it out. However, with that in mind, jug style filters are a good start.

However, many countries around the world also add fluoride to their tap water. Jug style water filters unfortunately do not remove fluoride. Personally, I would like to make my own decision about supplementing my diet with fluoride, thank you very much! I would strongly object to having it sneaked into my drinking water without my consent, as various negative health consequences have been reported, including disturbing our blood sugar homeostasis and encouraging insulin resistance (Lombarte et al. J Endocrinol. 2013).

The most complete way to achieve the purest water possible (including removal of all fluoride) is steam distillation using a water distiller. This is purer than any bottled or tap water and more effective than any other type of filtration. Of course, because water distillation is so complete, it naturally also removes all minerals from the tap water. There has been some debate as to whether the removal of minerals with water distillation leads to mineral deficiencies. The truth is that only 5 to 10% of our mineral intake actually comes from water. Distilling your own water (if fluoride is added) is a decision you have to make for yourself but as long your food provides enough minerals, I wouldn't worry about mineral deficiences.

Tea
Unsweetened green or white tea is great for our skin and for our

general health. I cannot praise these highly enough and I start every day with them. I also drink three to five mugs of green or white tea during the day. So the key question in this section is: how does a green or white tea bag turn water into an anti-aging elixir?

Green tea only contains minimal caffeine, but maximum flavonoids (catechins, a common group of polyphenolic compounds). These are known to have antioxidant, anti-inflammatory, anti-cancer and anti-aging effects (and also help with weight loss). These effects are highly beneficial to our skin and have been shown to reduce the sun's harmful effects (Rhodes et al. Br J Nutr. 2013).

A 12 week placebo-controlled study confirmed that drinking green tea can not only provide sun protection and increase blood flow and oxygen delivery into the skin, but even improve skin elasticity and roughness, thus improving overall skin quality (Heinrich et al. J Nutr. 2011). The anti-aging effects of green tea consumption on skin have also been well documented (Pazyar et al. Skinmed. 2012).

In a study by Fortes and coworker, it was even shown that daily tea drinking is protective for the most dangerous form of skin cancer, melanoma (Fortes et al. Int J Epidemiol. 2008). Tea-based catechins are also associated with longer telomeres (Fossel et al. John Wiley & Sons Inc. 2011).

White tea is similar to green tea, both are made from leaves of the tea plant Camellia sinensis. However, white tea leaves are picked very young, when the buds are still fresh and tender. At this point, the buds are covered in very fine, white hairs, which give white tea its name. White tea leaves are dried very gently, which maintains higher levels of antioxidants, while yielding less caffeine than other tea types.

Green and white teas are both highly beneficial to our skin and longevity and we should drinks lots and lots of them (of course unsweetened!). You can also buy green and white tea with flavoring. My favorites are 'White tea with Cherry Blossom', 'White tea with Elderflower & Apricot' and 'Green tea with Mango & Lychee' flavor. When preparing green and white tea, avoid pouring boiling water over the tea bag as this greatly reduces the heat-sensitive antioxidants. Let the water cool for a few minutes before pouring it over the leaves.

Other unsweetened herbal teas, fresh mint tea and the occasional black tea are fine also.

Coffee

While teas are all good, the data on coffee are controversial. Coffee contains a good level of antioxidants, but it is much higher in caffeine compared to all teas. Caffeine can raise stress hormone levels, which has a negative impact on our skin. The reported positive influences of coffee seem to come mainly from its antioxidant polyphenols. However, we can get these from green and white tea without the high caffeine content. As a result, I currently advise treating coffee as an occasional indulgence.

Coffee is also highly addictive. When I stopped drinking coffee a few years ago (for health reasons), I experienced a few very unpleasant days with flu-like withdrawal symptoms. I was convinced I must be coming down with something but, it turned out, I wasn't. It was simply coffee withdrawal and it settled after a few days. I believe it cannot be good to ingest something on a daily basis that makes you dependent on it!

Cocoa

Cocoa is very high in antioxidants (cocoa flavanols), which are very beneficial for our skin (Lee et al. J Agric Food Chem. 2003). However, when you drink cocoa, it is important to ensure that you use high quality, unsweetened 'real' cocoa and not the sugary instant variety. The importance of the quality of the cocoa beans and gentle processing was confirmed by a study we performed a few years ago. In our study, we looked at the antioxidant effects of flavanol-rich dark chocolate (Williams et al. J Cosmet Dermatol. 2009). Our study demonstrated that regular consumption of a chocolate particularly rich in flavanols can protect our skin from harmful UV effects. Conventional chocolate, however, had no such effect, because the high antioxidant capacity of fresh cocoa beans is often greatly reduced during the manufacturing process.

A different 12 week study confirmed that women who consumed a high flavanol cocoa drink benefited not only from reduced sun sensitivity, but also showed a measurably better blood flow in the skin, increased skin hydration, decreased skin roughness and improved skin thickness (Heinrich et al. J Nutr. 2006).

Alcohol

Some studies have found that light to moderate alcohol consumption can have some health benefits, including reduced cardiovascular mortality (Thompson et al. Med J Aust. 2013). In my opinion, the final jury is still out on this as there are a number of undeniable problems associated with drinking alcohol.

Alcohol (ethanol) consumption has been shown to increase oxidative stress and the highly reactive metabolite acetaldehyde is a key driver (McCarty. Med Hypotheses. 2013). Chronic alcohol consumption also leads to mitochondrial dysfunction (remember, mitochondria are the power houses of our cells) via generation of reactive oxygen species (ROS) and reactive nitrogen species (RNS).

Alcohol also ages us, an effect that can be partly explained by its stimulation of cortisol secretion, which of course accelerates aging. Excess alcohol intake has also been shown to shorten telomeres (Fyhrquist et al. Ann Med. 2012). By the way, alcohol is essentially a carbohydrate and most alcoholic beverages also contain added sugar and have a high GI (think alco-pops and cocktails).

Binge drinking seems particularly harmful and these episodes age you unbelievably! But it doesn't stop there. Alcohol consumption has even been shown to make your breasts look less attractive (Soltanian et al. Aesthet Surg J. 2012)! If that's not enough to stop you from drinking ...

So, in my opinion, it is best not to have alcohol too regularly and to always avoid over-indulging. However, if you do have some occasionally, I recommend a dry red wine. It contains the anti-aging 'miracle' compound resveratrol and a number of polyphenolic constituents plus its carbohydrate content is low. I have to admit that I am partial to the occasional glass of red wine myself.

What about fruit juice?

If eating fruit is healthy, surely drinking fruit juice must be too, correct? Actually no! Fruit juice is very high in sugar; you may as well drink sugar water. Even if it says '100% no sugar added', it still contains lots of fruit sugar (fructose) derived from the fruit itself and can be higher than the sugar content of sweet soft drinks. And remember that fructose is more active in AGE (Advanced Glycation End product) formation than glucose!

So, while it's fine to have whole fruits in moderation, because they contain fiber and have a much lower GI, you should avoid drinking fruit juices, even home-pressed ones. And the same goes for smoothies! Something that is always promoted as particularly healthy is also vegetable juice, for example, carrot juice. Vegetable juice also has a much higher GI than the whole vegetable and I would advise against it. Or at least limit intake – better to have the whole vegetable instead!

Sodas and sugary soft drinks

Sweetened sodas, lemonades and cola drinks should be avoided. Consumption of flavored, calorie-sweetened beverages has continued to play a major role in the epidemic of obesity, diabetes and fatty liver disease. It has even been named as a "threat to global health" (Popkin. Trends Endocrinol Metab. 2012).

Switching from cane sugar and fructose-laden beverages to low-calorie drinks containing artificial sweeteners such as aspartame and cyclamate is not recommended either, as we already discussed in the chapter on sugar. Instead, it is best to wean yourself off sweetened drinks completely and have water or unsweetened green or white tea instead. By the way, adding a little freshly squeezed lime or lemon, plus some fresh mint leaves, to your water (hot, lukewarm or cold) makes a lovely, refreshing drink. This is what I drink every day in addition to my green and white tea.

Remember ...
- Drink lots of water and unsweetened teas
- Green and white tea are particularly beneficial for our skin
- Avoid any sweetened (both sugar- and sweetener-based) beverages
- Avoid fruit juices, smoothies and vegetable juices!
- Coffee and red wine are fine on occasions

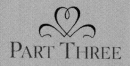

PART THREE

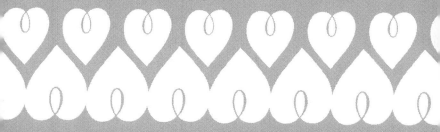

Chapter 10

Back to basics

So, having learned about keeping to a diet free of sugar and grain based foods, you may be thinking, "Am I going to be in permanent ketosis?" The answer is no. You may occasionally dip in and out of mild ketosis, but it won't be for any significant length of time. The amount of carbohydrates provided by vegetables, fruit, nuts and some starchy tubers will prevent that. But your body's metabolism will still be optimized, with a reduction in inflammation, glycation and oxidative stress.

For those of you who are unsure about ketosis and ketone bodies, let me explain briefly. Ketone bodies are produced as by-products when fat is broken down for energy generation. Occasional nutritional ketosis is a completely natural physiological reaction. Mild nutritional ketosis is beneficial in many ways. For example, it can increase glutathione levels (our 'master-antioxidant') and protect our DNA and mitochondria (Milder et al. Epilepsy Res. 2012). Ketone bodies have also been shown to be protective by reducing cell death, oxidative stress and free radical production (Haces et al. Exp Neurol. 2008). For those reasons a ketogenic diet is used successfully in many patients with treatment-resistant epilepsy (Milder et al. Epilepsy Res. 2012).

Before the advent of grain agriculture, our bodies would have been dipping in and out of nutritional ketosis frequently as part of its normal metabolism. However, as our modern Western diet is now so high in carbohydrate intake, the harmless and well-regulated nutritional ketosis is rarely experienced these days. Consequently, many people and even doctors mistake mild nutritional ketosis for pathological diabetic ketoacidosis, which is a harmful stress reaction occurring in diabetes patients. Let me reassure you, occasional mild nutritional ketosis is a completely normal, harmless and, in many ways, beneficial reaction that our body is perfectly equipped to deal with.

And you don't need to worry about the infamous ketosis 'grape-breath'. Even if you occasionally dip in and out of mild ketosis, once your body has learned to use ketone bodies efficiently, it will be able to generate and use them effectively without having to excrete acetone leftovers via your breath.

Is this Atkins?
I am often asked whether the Future Food Plan™ is a type of Atkins diet. The answer is a clear no. In the Atkins diet, you cut down carbohydrates much more radically and may even have to restrict your intake of vegetables to meet that target. There also seems to be no emphasis on eating high quality, whole foods and optimizing your omega-6/-3 ratio in the Atkins diet. So for all I know, you may be eating

processed foods all day long. In fact they even sell their own range of processed foods and snack bars.

With the Future Food Plan™, we are going back to basics and eating the way our body is designed to eat (I will talk more about this in the next chapter) – a highly nourishing and healthy, long-term way of eating, ideal for both skin health and longevity.

CHAPTER 11

If it comes in a wrapper

Convenience & processed foods

You now know all the basics about which foods are best and which should be avoided to maintain your skin in a beautiful, youthful condition and maximize your potential life span. Well done!

I now want to talk a little about food preparation. In general, we should try to eat whole foods in their most natural state as much as possible. Whole foods are those that are complete, i.e. not processed or refined. Avoiding all processed and re-fined foods, all fast food and ready meals is arguably one of the most important tips in this book. I cannot stress enough how fundamentally crucial this is.

Eating whole foods limits our intake of unnecessary additives and industrially-modified, poor-quality ingredients, and brings our diet closer to that which our bodies are designed to con-sume. Most of the pre-packaged, processed food in our super-markets these days contains unwelcome ingredients such as sugar, HFC syrup, soy protein, modified starches and polyunsaturated vegetable oils. Some of what we find on the super-market shelves I would not even call real food; it is best de-scribed as an industrial concoction. Processing of foods will also greatly increase the amount of external AGEs you take in with your food!

So in summary, if it comes in a wrapper or some other pack-aging – think again and check the label! Instead of buying processed and convenience foods, stick to fresh vegetables, fish, meat, eggs, nuts and fruit and prepare the meal yourself.

Preparing foods at home

I have already mentioned the problem of increased AGEs present in processed foods, however, it is also possible to acci-dentally increase the level of AGEs in your home-cooked food. For example, foods that are prepared at high temperatures, or been overcooked or over-browned, will generally contain more AGEs. Browning of food causes a so-called 'maillard reaction', which is associated with chronic complications of aging and age-related diseases (Edeas et al. Pathol Biol (Paris). 2010).

So my advice is to prepare your food as gently as possible and avoid very high temperatures and over-browning where possi-ble. I understand that you can't slow cook all your food but, in general, it is important to know the background. The worst possible kind of preparation is to burn your food or eat it in a 'charcoaled' state – so no typical English BBQ any longer I am afraid!

Organic or not organic?

If possible, I would buy certified organic foods as they are produced without synthetic compounds such as pesticides, herbicides and fertilizers, hormones, irradiation, industrial solvents and chemical additives. I would rather not have any of these in my food.

However, there are certain foods which are more important to buy as organic produce than others. These include foods with large surface areas, such as leafy green vegetables including spinach, rocket and kale. Vegetables and fruit with soft, edible skins, such as berries, apples and peppers, that are eaten as whole, i.e. not peeled, are also good to buy as organic produce. For food items with hard, inedible skins, for example, nuts, avocado or melon, which you peel, it is not quite so important. This is just general guidance and not set in stone. Ideally, buy whatever you can as organic produce.

Personally, I also prefer buying organic meat. I was really shocked when I first roasted an organic chicken and saw the difference. Compared to a 'normal' chicken, the consistency of the meat was completely different and there was also far less of it, making me wonder what had been done to the poor non-organic chicken to make it 'blow up' in that way.

But don't forget, organic is not the be all and end all. Just because it says organic on the label, does not always mean it is good. Think about organic cane sugar or organic refined wheat flour. So let common sense prevail.

How does this work in everyday life?
The great thing about this way of eating is that it's not about deprivation and hardship at all. You will enjoy plenty of tasty,

rich, natural foods. There will be no need to restrict yourself to dry, low-fat foods any longer. You can throw away the low-fat shackles!

Yes, you will need to allow more time to plan and prepare food, as sandwiches from the convenience store are now off the menu. But it also means that you can get into cooking, if you are not already. I understand that not everyone loves cooking. In fact, I hate cooking (there you go, I said it...). I know as a woman and mother I am supposed to enjoy it, or at least pretend that I do, but I just don't. So my husband and I usually take turns, because we know how important it is for long-term health. It's simply one of those things. You may not enjoy it, but it has to be done.

The great news is that there are so many adjusted recipes available now, where skin-unfriendly favorites have been adjusted to fit in with this new, and more skin-healthy and anti-aging type of eating. Countless recipes can be found online and there are also some great recipe books around including Aglaée Jacob's 'Digestive Health with Real Food: The Cookbook'.

Going out

When going out to a restaurant, you can usually follow this way of eating quite easily. Simply choose a meal with some form of protein, either fish or meat, and add vegetables or a salad on the side instead of rice, pasta or potatoes. As a dessert, strawberries with cream or a fruit salad would be great options. Even real ice cream (not a low-fat sorbet!) is not a bad choice as a treat, as it is low in GI/GL. Or alternatively order a cheese board for dessert. Again, if attending a BBQ, go for the meat or fish plus salads, but pass on the offer of a bun. Of course you won't have 100% control over the exact ingredients, but don't forget, every little helps. Just go with the flow, keep the momentum going and make the right choices.

I really like going out actually, as it fits well with the Future Food Plan™. Indian restaurants are one of my favorites. I just leave the naan bread and rice to one side and have some of their wonderful vegetables side dishes instead. Our local Indian restaurant, where we often order a take-away for the family, even offers to prepare everything with olive oil for a very small added charge.

A couple of times per month or so, I may have a 'cheat day'. We may be invited for dinner or to an event, where I have little influence on what is served. One those occasions I genuinely enjoy the meal and don't feel guilty, as I know I will be going back to the Future Food Plan™ the next day.

Also in the 'Anti-aging rocket fuel' chapter I will share an amazing trick to help you back on track when you have fallen off the wagon. It will kick your metabolism back in shape in no time and 'neutralize' occasional sins. Read on!

Remember ...
- Try to eat whole foods in their most natural state
- Shun processed and convenience foods!
- Prepare your food as gently as possible
- Buy organic produce if you can

CHAPTER 12

Ditch the food pyramid

It is time for a recap. I would like you to eat lots and lots of vegetables (this should be the large base of our new, skin-healthy food pyramid), plenty of 'good' fats such as monounsaturated oils and medium chain saturated fats, and a good daily portion of protein in the form of fish, eggs and meat. You can also eat moderate amounts of nuts, fruit and starchy tubers. You should avoid sugar and all sugar-containing foods, all grain-based foods and legumes. And last, but not least, stay clear of all processed foods!

So let's create a new food pyramid, a skin-healthy and longevity-enhancing food pyramid that will keep your skin and whole body in top shape for decades to come! Remember we want to be ready when that exciting life-extending research comes to fruition.

Our Future Food Plan™ food pyramid:
1.) Eat lots and lots of:
 * Fibrous vegetables (abundant servings, ideally organic)
 * Herbs and spices to add flavor
 * Drink plenty of water and unsweetened green or white tea

2.) Eat plenty of:
Healthy fats, for example:
* Olive oil
* Macadamia nut oil
* Coconut oil
* Avocados and avocado oil

3.) Eat good amounts of:
High quality, non-processed protein daily:
* Fish (non-farmed)
* Meat (organic, from grass-fed animals)
* Eggs (ideally from pasture-fed chickens)

4.) Eat moderate amounts of:
* Low-sugar fruit such as berries (best) and pitted fruit, ideally organic (minimize high sugar fruit such as bananas, grapes, mangos and other sweet tropical fruits)
* Nuts (other than peanuts)
* Starchy tubers and root vegetables (e.g. sweet potato, yam, winter squash, butternut squash)
* Full fat, fermented dairy products (organic)
* Animal fats from meat, butter, ghee, full fat cream etc.

5.) Sensible Indulgences:
* 2–4 squares of dark chocolate (85% cocoa) on occasion
* A glass of dry red wine on occasion
* Coffee
* Unsweetened nut butters (other than peanut butter)

6.) Avoid as much as possible:
* All grains and grain-based foods, including bread, pasta, pasties, biscuits, cakes, etc. (unless baked with grain-free flour)
* Breakfast cereals, porridge and oats
* Other starch-based foods (e.g. rice, rice crackers, popcorn, potatoes, sweet corn, legumes etc.)
* Fruit juices and smoothies
* Dried fruit
* Alcohol (other than the occasional glass of red wine)

7.) Avoid:

* ✻ Sugar and sugar-containing foods
* ✻ Fructose-based sweeteners (including agave syrup, maple syrup and honey)
* ✻ Sweet soft drinks and fizzy drinks
* ✻ Artificial sweeteners
* ✻ Low-calorie, diet beverages
* ✻ Bad fats including trans fats, hydrogenated or partially hydrogenated fats and margarine
* ✻ All omega-6 rich vegetable oils including polyunsaturated sunflower oil, safflower oil, corn oil, canola oil etc.
* ✻ Chips and crisps
* ✻ All processed foods!!!

Figure 4: The Future Food Plan™ food pyramid – supporting superior skin health and longevity.

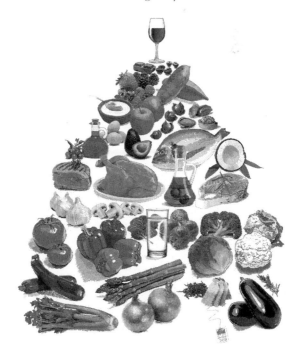

CHAPTER 13

Anti-aging rocket fuel

After all this, there is one more thing I want to share. It's true anti-aging rocket fuel and one of the best-kept secrets for longevity.

To maximize longevity and long-term health, it is not only important what you eat, but also when you eat it. No doubt your mum encouraged you to keep regular meal times. Well, it may come as a surprise to hear that de-regulating meal times can actually promote longevity.

Deregulating meal times simply means avoiding eating your meals at exactly the same time each day, but varying meal times at random. This is much more in keeping with how we are meant to eat and how, in fact, our primal ancestors arranged their meal times because circumstances forced them to eat more randomly. They simply ate whenever food was available, which wasn't as predictable as today with the availability of refrigeration and supermarkets. It was out of the question to have three set main meals, plus two snacks each day, which is the advice we receive today.

As I mentioned at the start, our genes haven't changed much since then and our body actually thrives on intermittent scarcity. It also allows it to deal more effectively with occasional excess!

Getting the timing right

So to future proof yourself further, I suggest to try and arrange your three meals at more irregular intervals and maybe even try skipping a meal on occasions. I know this goes against all current 'healthy' eating advice, but you should know by now, that official advice is not always correct, in fact, sometimes it can be plain wrong.

Irregular meal times keep your body guessing when the next food is going to arrive. This 'uncertainty' leads your body to avoid wasting precious resources and try and look after and repair whatever it can, which requires less energy. So, instead of relentlessly dividing its cells like a mad man on a spending spree, your body becomes more resourceful and looks after what it has while wasting as little as possible. This all encourages cell repair.

It is also beneficial for anti-aging purposes to not eat after 7pm (other than a small protein snack, if need be), as this will encourage HGH (our 'Youth Hormone') release at night.

Always on the go

Have you ever thought about the consequences of multi-tasking and eating on the run? Sitting in front of the TV for dinner, munching at your desk while checking emails or eating a quick sandwich while walking or driving to your next appointment? That's not a good idea! You can have the best diet in the world, but if you don't sit down properly to eat, chew thoroughly and enjoy your meal slowly, you may not be digesting the food as well as you could. This could lead to suboptimal resorption of nutrients needed for skin health and longevity.

Try to turn meal times into a happy, relaxed social event if you can. Take the time to sit down at a table, enjoy the smells and eat mindfully, in order to get saliva production and stomach acid going. We need our parasympathetic nervous system switched on to digest our food properly and this happens best if we are not stressed, distracted or on the run.

We are not supposed to behave like cows
We are also sometimes advised to 'graze' throughout the day and have five or as many as eight meals per day rather than three main meals. This 'grazing' idea is very much in vogue at the moment and I am sure you will have read the articles in glossy magazines. Unfortunately, this approach is not very good for skin health, general health and longevity. To find out why, let's look first at why we are advised to 'graze'.

The aim of 'grazing' throughout the day is to "keep your energy levels steady" and "avoid sugar lows". We all know that sugar lows can lead to low energy levels, food cravings and subsequent over-eating. However, this only happens in typical 'carbivores', where the body uses carbohydrates as its main fuel type. When following the Future Food Plan™, your body will be perfectly equipped and very happy to use alternative means of fuel, such as fat, which is always available.

But despite that, what's the problem with 'grazing' in the first place? Let's look at this again. We are advised to eat throughout the day to "avoid sugar lows", which suggests that we are supposed to keep our sugar levels high throughout the entire day! If you have learned nothing else in this book, I hope you now understand that high blood sugar levels make us age at lightning speed. The higher the average blood sugar level, the quicker we age. It is as simple as that. So to keep blood sugar and insulin levels, oxidative stress, glycation and inflammation processes down, we should avoid grazing.

Snacking randomly throughout the day has also been shown to decrease insulin sensitivity. In a remarkable study published in 2011, it was shown that animals snacking on a typical human cafeteria diet experienced a dramatic increase in body weight (much more than the animals on a normal high fat diet) as well as a decrease in insulin sensitivity, with spikes in glucose and insulin levels. The snacking animal group also displayed remarkable systemic inflammation compared to the traditional high fat diet of the control group (Sampey et al. Obesity (Silver Spring). 2011).

The good news is that you will not need the 'crutch' of grazing if you have successfully changed your eating habits following the Future Food Plan™. High blood sugar levels are only needed to maintain energy levels if your body is dependent on sugar as its main energy source. After reprogramming your metabolism, your energy levels will remain perfectly steady all day, even with irregular meal times or skipping meals. Your body is using fat as its main energy source and this is plentiful at all times. So with the Future Food Plan™, you can slow down the aging process by keeping your blood sugar and insulin levels, with all their negative consequences, low without ever feeling hypoglycemic.

Caloric restriction for longevity?

You may have come across caloric restriction (CR) when reading about extending life span. Calorie restriction, which means limiting food and energy intake on an ongoing basis, is one of the best investigated strategies for delaying aging, deferring the onset of age-associated diseases and extending lifespan (Roth et al. Maturitas. 2012; Ribaric. Oxid Med Cell Longev. 2012; Tucci. Aging (Albany NY). 2012; Pallauf et al. Ageing Res Rev. 2012).

CR has also been shown to prevent or delay aging-related changes in our skin and increase the density of fibroblasts and our skin's connective tissue fibers collagen and elastin (Bhattacharyya et al. Arch Facial Plast Surg. 2005). Many of CR's positive effects on longevity are achieved via induction of Sirtuin 1 (SIRT1), a member of the sirtuin family of proteins, which are important for cellular regulation. Studies have also confirmed that CR induces changes in hormone levels, including an increase in some of our natural youth hormones (e.g. HGH and DHEA) and a decrease in IGF-1. These CR-induced endocrine changes result in a decline in pathologies and increased life span (Sonntag et al. J Gerontol A Biol Sci Med Sci. 1999).

There is now a whole worldwide movement of devoted people restricting their calorie intake on a daily basis, in order to increase longevity and long-term health. To be honest, while CR may make theoretical sense, I wouldn't want to live in such misery. But here is some great news! You can mimic many of the beneficial effects of CR (including SIRT1 induction) with moderation of carbohydrate intake and insulin release (Blüher et al. Science. 2003, Klöting et al. Exp Gerontol. 2005).

IF – the best kept secret to increased longevity

But now let me tell you the best-kept anti-aging secret of all. If you want to really boost your anti-aging efforts in a much easier way than daily caloric restriction, try intermittent fasting, also known as IF (Honjoh et al. Nature. 2009). I am a big fan and so is my husband; it seems to suit men just as well.

Essentially, IF is an enhanced version of deregulating meal times and there are different ways of doing it. For example, one way is to alternate days of fast and feast. The way I find most practical though is to fast for 24 hours twice each week. One way of doing this is to avoid eating from dinner the previous day until dinner the next day (i.e. skip breakfast and lunch). It doesn't necessarily have to be from dinner to dinner, but that's simply what I like to do. If you prefer breakfast to breakfast, or lunch to lunch, that is fine also. During this time, you can still drink lots of water and unsweetened teas, but must avoid eating any food.

What are the benefits of IF? Like deregulated meal times, but to a greater extent, it kicks your body into thinking the good times are over. It stops 'burning the candle at both ends' and becomes sensible, optimizing cell repair instead of wasting energy. There is a sophisticated mechanism called autophagy, a cellular process where each cell gets rid of any problematic content. This not only applies to infectious agents such as bacteria and viruses, but also to toxic waste or its own damaged, malformed or dysfunctional cell components. Autophagy also ensures the turnover of aged components. When digesting this cellular junk, it is broken down into its constituent parts, such as fatty acids, amino acids and sugar. These can then be reused by the cell – a true recycling process.

Cells try to keep levels of fatty acids, amino acids and sugars constant, so when these become readily available with our food, autophagy is suppressed (Jaminet. Simon & Schuster. 2012). When levels become scarce, however, autophagy is increased (Galluzzi et al. Biochem Soc Trans. 2008). That means that when fasting, our cells ramp up the process of tidying up, because they are trying to find cellular junk they can dismantle in order to obtain building blocks needed. Without autophagy, our cells cannot survive. Fairly recently, a study demonstrated that promoting autophagy can extend lifespan by as much as 50% (Vellai. Cell Death Differ. 2009). Intermittent fasting promotes healthy autophagy.

Intermittent fasting has also been shown to increase insulin sensitivity and glucose uptake and decrease oxidative damage in our body. During fasting, secretion of human growth hormone (HGH), our 'youth hormone', also increases in a natural way. However, as certain tissues become less sensitive to HGH stimulation, we find a reduced induction of IGF-1 and other not so desirable growth factors. Intermittent fasting has even been found to protect our brain cells and reduce the risk of dementia (Anson et al. Proc Natl Acad Sci U S A. 2003; Halagappa et al. Neurobiol Dis. 2007).

Intermittent fasting also improves immune function. I often wonder whether nature takes away our appetite deliberately when we are threatened by some illness in order to fight it more effectively. Lastly, IF is amazingly helpful for weight management. And most reassuring is that the benefits are not lost if you eat more than usual the next day.

Are you worried about whether you can make it through 24 hours without any food? Well, 24 hours is not actually that long considering you will be sleeping a third of that time. Also, your body is already used to dealing with fasting periods, as it does a 10- to 12-hour fast every single night. So don't worry, you will be able to do it. And don't forget hunger does not keep building up. You may notice it initially, but then it's gone again five or ten minutes later. It might come and go in gentle waves, but much less than you might fear.

Let me also reassure you that, if you have been following my advice regarding moderating carbohydrate intake and insulin release, you are very likely to find IF surprisingly easy. A typical 'carbivore' may find it difficult due to the repeated sugar-highs and sugar-lows throughout a normal day and their body's reliance on glucose as primary fuel. Your body however, will be fully trained to comfortably use fat as primary fuel source and therefore will not feel too much different when fasting.

If you don't take my word for it, just try it! Trust me, if you are adapted to the Future Food Plan™ you will not suffer with hypoglycemic energy lows while fasting. You will be able to fast easily and effortlessly and may even find it somewhat elevating. If, however, you feel slightly light-headed at any point, which is likely caused by lack of salt intake while fasting, some homemade bone broth will ameliorate this quickly. Homemade bone broth is a great thing to have stock-frozen for other occasions anyway, as it is very rich in minerals and glycosaminoglycans (GAGs).

I suggest starting trying IF once you have been on the Future Food Plan™ for around three weeks as it makes sense to reprogram your metabolism first. You can do it straight away if you prefer the tough approach but it may just be a little bit trickier. But, even if IF is the only thing you take away from this book, it will still make a massive difference.

Getting back on track

Intermittent fasting is also an ideal way to kick your metabolic function back into shape if you have gone off track for some reason. So, after a party with lots of processed carbohydrates or an indulgent weekend away, try doing a 24 hours fast to 'neutralize' some of the negative consequences of that indulgence. Another way to support your metabolism if you have had a carb-infused meal is to go for a walk (or dance!), as this improves insulin sensitivity and diverts some of the ingested glucose straight into your muscles, allowing them to burn it away.

Remember ...
- Avoid 'grazing'
- Try deregulating your meal times
- Play around with intermittent fasting to improve cellular function and support longevity (e.g. two 24 hour fasts per week)
- Physical activity after a meal improves insulin sensitivity

---

A quick recap!

By adapting to the Future Food Plan™ you will lay down one of the most important corner stones for a long and healthy life, and look beautiful all the way! It has countless benefits including:

- Enhanced cellular and immune function
- Optimized repair of cells
- Improved antioxidant capacity and reduced oxidative stress
- Reduced inflammation
- Reduced glycation
- Stabilized appetite and energy levels
- Optimized fat metabolism and weight management
- Reduced risk factors for many modern diseases including diabetes, cardiovascular disease and cancers
- Delayed aging processes and increased longevity

It really is worth the effort because you will feel so much better, believe me! What is your health and longevity worth? What are you worth? This is an important investment that will pay massive health dividends in the long run.

However, while nutrition is a vital component, there are other lifestyle habits that are equally important to future proof your skin and support longevity. There is not enough space to cover everything in this particular book. My next book focuses on all the other things you can do to future proof your skin and support longevity on a daily basis. There continues to be a lot of misinformation out there so stay tuned, I will be back with the latest scientific research!

In summary, I have presented you with the optimal way of eating to future proof your skin and your body and, of course, I would love you to fully adapt to the Future Food Plan™. However, even if you decide not to take it all on board and follow only selected recommendations to start with, every small change in the right direction is worth doing. And with time, I am sure you will be taking on more and more of the recommendations as you start seeing and feeling the changes.

Start future proofing yourself – today!

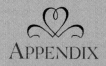

APPENDIX

Future Food Plan™ Sample Menu

Monday

Breakfast:
Greek yoghurt (full fat with live cultures) with blueberries, macadamia nut halves and a sprinkle of raw cocoa nibs.
Green tea.

Lunch:
Chicken salad: Cold chicken from previous day's Sunday roast. Serve with a pile of rocket salad, cherry tomatoes and shavings of Parmesan cheese, generous drizzle of olive oil and some balsamic vinegar.
Berry-coconut 'smoothie' (coconut milk, mixed berries, unsweetened vanilla powder).

Dinner:
Duck and kale: Roast duck breast with rosemary sprigs and garlic butter. Serve with a large pile of steamed kale with a generous drizzle of macadamia nut oil.
Skin friendly, oat- and grain-free chocolate flapjack for dessert.

Tuesday

Breakfast:
Large mushroom and spring onion omelet.
White tea with cherry blossom flavor.

Lunch:
Gazpacho starter: Mix raw red pepper, a tin of tomatoes, half a cucumber, quarter of an onion, a clove of garlic, a pinch of salt, some olive oil and a tablespoon of red wine vinegar in a blender. Serve cold.
Large pile of cold green asparagus spears (drizzled in lemon and plenty of olive oil, sprinkled with pine nuts and a little salt) with cold slices of roast turkey.

| **Dinner:** | Trout with almonds and okra: Cook a fillet of trout gently in pure virgin coconut oil and a handful of flaked almonds. Serve with a large portion of stir-fried okra and tomatoes with a sprinkle of turmeric.
Strawberries with cream for dessert. |

Wednesday

Breakfast:	Hot, oat-less porridge: Unsweetened almond milk with three tablespoons of ground mixed nuts (kitchen blender) and two tablespoons of unsweetened coconut flakes. Heat in microwave. Sprinkle with ground cinnamon and a handful of berries (or grate an apple with skin into the mixture). Fresh mint tea.
Lunch:	Avocado and sweet potato salad with crab meat: Slices of cucumber and tomatoes, green beans, black olives, one avocado and half a boiled sweet potato, cut into cubes. Add crabmeat to optimize your daily protein quota. Drizzle generously with avocado oil and add some lemon juice.
Dinner:	'Shakshuka' peppers and poached egg: Fry red onion, green, red and yellow peppers gently in pure virgin coconut oil with half a tin of tomatoes and some eggplant (aubergine) cubes, simmered for half an hour. Add half teaspoon of turmeric and few strands of saffron, then break a few eggs into the mixture. Put the lid on and leave until the white is set. A few squares of 85% dark chocolate for dessert.

Thursday

| **Breakfast:** | Slices of smoked salmon with a ripe sliced avocado, black pepper and a squeeze of lemon.
Hot chocolate: heat a mix of unsweetened almond milk, cocoa powder, some fresh mint leaves and a little stevia/erythritol sweetener. |

Lunch: Tinned sardines with homemade coleslaw: Finely-slice red & white cabbage, red onion and some apple. Mix with plain, full-fat yoghurt, squeezed lemon and crushed garlic. Scatter with pumpkin seeds. Cheese for dessert.

Dinner: Steak, 'fries' and salad: Buffalo steak with large, mixed green salad with homemade vinaigrette dressing. Plenty of aubergine (eggplant) 'French fries' on the side. Cherries for dessert.

Friday

Breakfast: Large, plain, unsweetened coconut yoghurt with chopped mixed nuts, half-teaspoon cinnamon and a handful of raspberries.
White tea with Elderflower flavor.

Lunch: Large portion of raw carrot sticks, whole radishes and celery with homemade lamb's liver pate.
Skin-friendly, homemade carrot cake for dessert.

Dinner: Ground pecan encrusted wild Alaskan salmon. Serve with lots of steamed broccoli with a knob of butter and some gently boiled sweet potato on the side.
A glass of dry red wine.

Saturday

Breakfast: Scrambled eggs with a crumble of feta cheese and wilted spinach. Hot lime drink (squeeze of fresh lime with some fresh mint leaves in hot water).

Lunch: Asian seafood stir-fry: Stir-fry a selection of rainbow-colored chopped vegetables (e.g. red peppers, zucchini (courgettes), leek) with mixed seafood and a little ginger and garlic. Cook all the ingredients in pure virgin coconut oil. Serve with cauliflower 'rice' (grated cauliflower, very briefly fried in macadamia nut oil).

| **Dinner:** | Minced lamb 'Bolognaise' sauce with fresh thyme served with a large pile of greens and a small portion of gently boiled winter nut squash on the side.

Homemade, skin friendly blueberry & strawberry 'crips'/'crumble' for dessert. |

Sunday

| **Breakfast:** | Plain, full-fat, fermented kefir drink, pistachio nuts and a ripe peach. |

| **Lunch:** | Sunday roast: Roast chicken in sage, scattered garlic cloves and red onions. Serve with boiled Brussels sprouts with butter. Large portion of cauliflower mash on the side. |

| **Dinner:** | Creamy Clam Chowder Soup, made with homemade chicken stock.

Homemade forest berries ice-cream with almond flakes for dessert. |

Future Food Plan™ Shopping Essentials

- MUFA rich oils, for example macadamia nut oil, extra virgin olive oil and avocado oil
- Virgin coconut oil
- Mixed nuts, for example, macadamia nuts, pecans, almonds and pistachios
- Coconut flour and blanched almond flour
- Ground almonds
- A skin friendly sweetener such as a stevia/erythritol mix or 100% birch wood derived xylitol
- Organic, unsweetened cocoa powder
- Eggs
- Full-fat, live Greek Yoghurt
- Lots of fresh and frozen vegetables
- Fresh and frozen berries
- Fish and meat, as needed

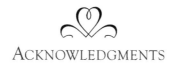

ACKNOWLEDGMENTS

I thank my husband Jay for the never-ending support he has given me throughout the long journey of writing this book.

I thank my children Elias, Cyrus and Kaia for being patient with me and allowing me to write on so many occasions.

I thank Tash and Matt for their encouragement – the bet is still on!

I thank Raymond Aaron and his team for giving me the push to go ahead and write this book.

I thank my graphic designers Rodrigo Hernández Artiach and Budi Saputra for their great work on layout, graphics and book cover.

I thank Lynn Hamilton for her amazing editorial assistance and Ruth Kerr for thorough proof reading.

ABOUT THE AUTHOR

Dr Stefanie Williams is a fully qualified medical doctor and specialist dermatologist. She is founder and medical director at European Dermatology London (www.eudelo.com), a renowned private skin clinic in London.

Dr Stefanie graduated in Medicine in Germany. After many years of post-graduate specialist training and success in the rigorous German specialization exam, she was awarded the title of Specialist in Dermatology by the Hamburg Medical Council. Dr Stefanie has gained extensive clinical experience in both Germany and Great Britain and has undertaken research in a number of European University departments. In her London-based skin clinic, she not only treats the entire spectrum of skin diseases and troubled skin, but also practises cosmetic dermatology, ensuring the highest quality and safety standards. As a medical doctor, a dermatologist and a cosmetic scientist, Dr Stefanie is in a unique position to combine her in-depth knowledge of skin biology with her expertise in anti-aging medicine, prevention and skincare.

Dr Stefanie is author and co-author of more than 100 scientific articles, book chapters and abstracts and is frequently asked to speak at international conferences. She lectures in the Division of Cosmetic Science at the University of the Arts, London. Dr Stefanie is often quoted as an expert in glossy magazines and newspapers and has appeared on TV as a skin expert.

Dr Stefanie lives with her husband and three children in South-West London.

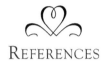

REFERENCES

* Adebamowo C, Spiegelman D, Berkey C, et al. Milk consumption and acne in teenaged boys. J Am Acad Dermatol. 2008;58(5):787-93.

* Anlasik T, Sies H, Griffiths HR, et al. Dietary habits are major determinants of the plasma antioxidant status in healthy elderly subjects. Br J Nutr. 2005;94(5):639-42.

* Amarasiri WA, Dissanayake AS. Coconut fats. Ceylon Med J. 2006;51(2):47-51.

* Anson RM, Guo Z, de Cabo R, et al. Intermittent fasting dissociates beneficial effects of dietary restriction on glucose metabolism and neuronal resistance to injury from calorie intake. Proc Natl Acad Sci USA. 2003;100(10):6216-20.

* Anunciato TP, da Rocha Filho PA. Carotenoids and polyphenols in nutricosmetics, nutraceuticals, and cosmeceuticals. J Cosmet Dermatol. 2012;11(1):51-4.

* Austin MA, Hokanson JE, Edwards KL. Hypertriglyceridemia as a cardiovascular risk factor. Am J Cardiol. 1998; 81(4A):7B-12B.

* Avery NC, Bailey AJ. The effects of the Maillard reaction on the physical properties and cell interactions of collagen. Pathol Biol (Paris). 2006;54(7):387-95.

* Bakke-McKellep AM, Koppang EO, Gunnes G, et al. Histological, digestive, metabolic, hormonal and some immune factor responses in Atlantic salmon, Salmo salar L., fed genetically modified soybeans. J Fish Dis. 2007;30(2):65-79.

* Bartke A. Minireview: role of the growth hormone/insulin-like growth factor system in mammalian aging. Endocrinology. 2005;146(9):3718-23.

* Bates GW. Body weight control practice as a cause of infertility. Clin Obstet Gynecol. 1985;28(3):632-44.

* Bhattacharyya TK, Merz M, Thomas JR. Modulation of cutaneous aging with calorie restriction in Fischer 344 rats: a histological study. Arch Facial Plast Surg. 2005;7(1):12-6.

* Blesso CN, Andersen CJ, Barona J, et al. Whole egg consumption improves lipoprotein profiles and insulin sensitivity to a greater extent than yolk-free egg substitute in individuals with metabolic syndrome. Metabolism. 2013;62(3):400-10.

* Blesso CN, Andersen CJ, Bolling BW, Fernandez ML. Egg intake improves carotenoid status by increasing plasma HDL cholesterol in adults with metabolic syndrome. Food Funct. 2013;4(2):213-21.

* Blüher M, Kahn BB, Kahn CR. Extended longevity in mice lacking the insulin receptor in adipose tissue. Science. 2003;299(5606):572-4.

* Bouilly-Gauthier D, Jeannes C, Maubert Y, et al. Clinical evidence of benefits of a dietary supplement containing probiotic and carotenoids on ultraviolet-induced skin damage. Br J Dermatol. 2010;163(3):536-43.

* Boukamp P. Skin aging: a role for telomerase and telomere dynamics? Curr Mol Med. 2005;5(2):171-7.

∗ Buckingham EM, Klingelhutz AJ. The role of telomeres in the ageing of human skin. Exp Dermatol. 2011;20(4):297-302.

∗ Calvo E, Luu-The V, Morissette J, et al. Pangenomic changes induced by DHEA in the skin of postmenopausal women. J Steroid Biochem Mol Biol. 2008;112(4-5):186-93.

∗ Cicerale S, Lucas LJ, Keast RS. Antimicrobial, antioxidant and anti-inflammatory phenolic activities in extra virgin olive oil. Curr Opin Biotechnol. 2012; 23(2):129-35.

∗ Cohen AE, Johnston CS. Almond ingestion at mealtime reduces postprandial glycemia and chronic ingestion reduces hemoglobin A(1c) in individuals with well-controlled type 2 diabetes mellitus. Metabolism. 2011;60(9):1312-7.

∗ Danby FW. Nutrition and aging skin: sugar and glycation. Clin Dermatol. 2010; 28(4):409-11.

∗ Da Luz PL, Favarato D, Faria-Neto JR Jr, et al. High Ratio of Triglycerides to HDL-Cholesterol Predicts Extensive Coronary Disease. Clinics (Sao Paulo). 2008;63(4):427-32.

∗ Davis W. Wheat Belly. Lose the wheat, lose the weight, and find your path back to health. Rodale; 2011.

∗ De Grey A, Rae M. Ending Aging: The Rejuvenation Breakthroughs That Could Reverse Human Aging in Our Lifetime. St. Martin's Griffin; 2008.

∗ Donaldson MS. Nutrition and cancer: a review of the evidence for an anti-cancer diet. Nutr J. 2004;20;3:19.

∗ Dreher ML. Pistachio nuts: composition and potential health benefits. Nutr Rev. 2012;70(4):234-40.

* Dreher ML, Davenport AJ. Hass avocado composition and potential health effects. Crit Rev Food Sci Nutr. 2013;53(7):738-50.

* Dussutour A, Simpson SJ. Ant workers die young and colonies collapse when fed a high-protein diet. Proc Biol Sci. 2012;279(1737):2402-8.

* Edeas M, Attaf D, Mailfert AS, Nasu M, Joubet R. Maillard reaction, mitochondria and oxidative stress: potential role of antioxidants. Pathol Biol (Paris). 2010;58(3):220-5.

* Ellis KA, Innocent G, Grove-White D, et al. Comparing the fatty acid composition of organic and conventional milk. J Dairy Sci. 2006;89(6):1938-50.

* Emmerson E, Hardman MJ. The role of estrogen deficiency in skin ageing and wound healing. Biogerontology. 2012;13(1):3-20.

* Epel ES, Lin J, Wilhelm FH, et al. Cell aging in relation to stress arousal and cardiovascular disease risk factors. Psychoneuroendocrinology. 2006;31(3):277-87.

* Falus A, Marton I, Borbényi E, et al. [The 2009 Nobel Prize in Medicine and its surprising message: lifestyle is associated with telomerase activity]. Orv Hetil. 2010;151(24):965-70.

* Fanson BG, Taylor PW. Protein:carbohydrate ratios explain life span patterns found in Queensland fruit fly on diets varying in yeast:sugar ratios. Age (Dordr). 2012;34(6):1361-8.

* Farzaneh-Far R, Lin J, Epel ES, et al. Association of marine omega-3 fatty acid levels with telomeric aging in patients with coronary heart disease. JAMA. 2010;303(3):250-7.

* Fernandez ML. Rethinking dietary cholesterol. Curr Opin Clin Nutr Metab Care. 2012;15(2):117-21.

∗ Fortes C, Mastroeni S, Melchi F, et al. A protective effect of the Mediterranean diet for cutaneous melanoma. Int J Epidemiol. 2008;37(5):1018-29.

∗ Fossel M, Blackburn G, Woynarowky D. The Immortality Edge. John Wiley & Sons Inc.; 2011.

∗ Foster-Powell K, Holt SHA, Brand-Miller JC. International table of glycemic index and glycemic load values: 2002. Am J Clin Nutr. 2002;76:5-56.

∗ Fulgoni VL 3rd, Dreher M, Davenport AJ. Avocado consumption is associated with better diet quality and nutrient intake, and lower metabolic syndrome risk in US adults: results from the National Health and Nutrition Examination Survey (NHANES) 2001-2008. Nutr J. 2013;12:1.

∗ Fyhrquist F, Saijonmaa O. Telomere length and cardiovascular aging. Ann Med. 2012;44 (Suppl 1):138-42.

∗ Galluzzi L, Morselli E, Vicencio JM, et al. Life, death and burial: multifaceted impact of autophagy. Biochem Soc Trans. 2008;36(Pt 5):786-90.

∗ Garg ML, Blake RJ, Wills RB, Clayton EH. Macadamia nut consumption modulates favourably risk factors for coronary artery disease in hypercholesterolemic subjects. Lipids. 2007;42(6):583-7.

∗ Geens T, Goeyens L, Covaci A. Are potential sources for human exposure to bisphenol-A overlooked? Int J Hyg Environ Health. 2011;214(5):339-47.

∗ Gibbs JC, Williams NI, Scheid JL, et al. The association of a high drive for thinness with energy deficiency and severe menstrual disturbances: confirmation in a large population of exercising women. Int J Sport Nutr Exerc Metab. 2011;21(4):280-90.

* Gilbert K, Arseneault-Bréard J, Flores Monaco F, et al. Attenuation of post-myocardial infarction depression in rats by n-3 fatty acids or probiotics starting after the onset of reperfusion. Br J Nutr. 2013;109(1):50-6.

* Gouranton E, Thabuis C, Riollet C, et al. Lycopene inhibits proinflammatory cytokine and chemokine expression in adipose tissue. J Nutr Biochem. 2011;22(7):642-8.

* Gruss C, Reed JA, Altmeyer P, et al. Induction of interstitial collagenase (MMP-1) by UVA-1 phototherapy in morphea fibroblasts. Lancet. 1997;350(9087):1295-6.

* Guéniche A, Philippe D, Bastien P, et al. Probiotics for photoprotection. Dermatoendocrinol. 2009;1(5):275-9.

* Gueniche A, Benyacoub J, Philippe D, et al. Lactobacillus paracasei CNCM I-2116 (ST11) inhibits substance P-induced skin inflammation and accelerates skin barrier function recovery in vitro. Eur J Dermatol. 2010;20(6):731-7.

* Gunn DA, de Craen AJ, Dick JL, et al. Facial appearance reflects human familial longevity and cardiovascular disease risk in healthy individuals. J Gerontol A Biol Sci Med Sci. 2013;68(2):145-52.

* Haces ML, Hernández-Fonseca K, Medina-Campos ON, et al. Antioxidant capacity contributes to protection of ketone bodies against oxidative damage induced during hypoglycemic conditions. Exp Neurol. 2008;211(1):85-96.

* Haffner SM, Stern MP, Hazuda HP, et al. Cardiovascular risk factors in confirmed prediabetic individuals. Does the clock for coronary heart disease start ticking before the onset of clinical diabetes? JAMA. 1990;263(21):2893-8.

* Halagappa VK, Guo Z, Pearson M, et al. Intermittent fasting and caloric restriction ameliorate age-related behavioral deficits in the triple-transgenic mouse model of Alzheimer's disease. Neurobiol Dis. 2007;26(1):212-20.

* Hayashi N, Togawa K, Yanagisawa M, et al. Effect of sunlight exposure and aging on skin surface lipids and urate. Exp Dermatol. 2003;12(Suppl 2):13-7.

* Heber D. Vegetables, fruits and phytoestrogens in the prevention of diseases. J Postgrad Med. 2004;50(2):145-9.

* He FJ, Marciniak M, Markandu ND, et al. Effect of modest salt reduction on skin capillary rarefaction in white, black, and Asian individuals with mild hypertension. Hypertension. 2010;56(2):253-9.

* Heinrich U, Neukam K, Tronnier H, et al. Long-term ingestion of high flavanol cocoa provides photoprotection against UV-induced erythema and improves skin condition in women. J Nutr. 2006;136(6):1565-9.

* Heinrich U, Moore CE, De Spirt S, et al. Green tea polyphenols provide photoprotection, increase microcirculation, and modulate skin properties of women. J Nutr. 2011;141(6):1202-8.

* Hong JW, Yang GE, Kim YB, et al. Anti-inflammatory activity of cinnamon water extract in vivo and in vitro LPS-induced models. BMC Complement Altern Med. 2012;12:237.

* Honjoh S, Yamamoto T, Uno M, Nishida E. Signalling through RHEB-1 mediates intermittent fasting-induced longevity in C. elegans. Nature. 2009;457(7230):726-30.

* Howgate DJ, Graham SM, Leonidou A, et al. Bone metabolism in anorexia nervosa: molecular pathways and current treatment modalities. Osteoporos Int. 2013;24(2):407-21.

* Jacobs DR Jr, Nettleton JA. Dietary intake of saturated fat by food source and incident cardiovascular disease: the Multi-Ethnic Study of Atherosclerosis. Am J Clin Nutr. 2012;96(2):397-404.

* Jaminet P, Jaminet SC. Perfect Health Diet. Simon & Schuster; 2012.

* Kang JX, Weylandt KH. Modulation of inflammatory cytokines by omega-3 fatty acids. Subcell Biochem. 2008;49:133-43.

* Kanter MM, Kris-Etherton PM, Fernandez ML, et al. Exploring the factors that affect blood cholesterol and heart disease risk: is dietary cholesterol as bad for you as history leads us to believe? Adv Nutr. 2012;3(5):711-7.

* Kiessling G, Schneider J, Jahreis G. Long-term consumption of fermented dairy products over 6 months increases HDL cholesterol. Eur J Clin Nutr. 2002;56(9):843-9.

* Kim J, Lim SY, Shin A, et al. Fatty fish and fish omega-3 fatty acid intakes decrease the breast cancer risk: a case-control study. BMC Cancer. 2009;9:216.

* Kimoto-Nira H, Suzuki C, Kobayashi M, et al. Anti-ageing effect of a lactococcal strain: analysis using senescence-accelerated mice. Br J Nutr. 2007;98(6):1178-86.

* Kleszczynski K, Fischer TW. Melatonin and human skin aging. Dermatoendocrinol. 2012; 4(3):245-52.

* Klöting N, Blüher M. Extended longevity and insulin signaling in adipose tissue. Exp Gerontol. 2005;40(11):878-83.

* Knuuttila ML, Kuoksa TH, Svanberg MJ, et al. Effects of dietary xylitol on collagen content and glycosylation in healthy and diabetic rats. Life Sci. 2000;67(3):283-90.

* Koshy JC et al. Effect of dietary zinc and phytase supplementation on botulinum toxin treatments. J Drugs Dermatol. 2012;11:507-12.

* Krutmann J. Pre- and probiotics for human skin. Clin Plast Surg. 2012;39(1):59-64.

* Kurzweil R, Grossman, T. Transcent. Nine steps to living well forever. Rodale; 2009.

* La Berge AF. How the Ideology of low-fat Conquered America. J Hist Med Allied Sci. 2008;63(2):139-77.

* Laron Z. Do deficiencies in growth hormone and insulin-like growth factor-1 (IGF-1) shorten or prolong longevity? Mech Ageing Dev. 2005;126(2):305-7.

* Latreille J, Kesse-Guyot E, Malvy D, et al. Dietary monounsaturated fatty acids intake and risk of skin photoaging. PLoS One. 2012;7(9):e44490.

* Lee KW, Kim YJ, Lee HJ, Lee CY. Cocoa has more phenolic phytochemicals and a higher antioxidant capacity than teas and red wine. J Agric Food Chem. 2003;51(25):7292-5.

* Liedo P, Carey JR, Ingram DK, Zou S. The interplay among dietary fat, sugar, protein and açai (Euterpe oleracea Mart.) pulp in modulating lifespan and reproduction in a Tephritid fruit fly. Exp Gerontol. 2012;47(7):536-9.

* Lima CF, Pereira-Wilson C, Rattan SI. Curcumin induces heme oxygenase-1 in normal human skin fibroblasts through redox signaling: relevance for anti-aging intervention. Mol Nutr Food Res. 2011;55(3):430-42.

* Liu C, Russell RM. Nutrition and gastric cancer risk: an update. Nutr Rev. 2008;66(5):237-49.

* Li XQ, Guo YY, De W. DNA methylation and microRNAs in cancer. World J Gastroenterol. 2012;18(9):882-8.

* Lombarte M, Fina BL, Lupo M, et al. Physical exercise ameliorates the toxic effect of fluoride on the insulin-glucose system. J Endocrinol. 2013;218(1):99-103.

* Lucas L, Russell A, Keast R. Molecular mechanisms of inflammation. Anti-inflammatory benefits of virgin olive oil and the phenolic compound oleocanthal. Curr Pharm Des. 2011;17(8):754-68.

* Maillot M, Drewnowski A. A conflict between nutritionally adequate diets and meeting the 2010 dietary guidelines for sodium. Am J Prev Med. 2012;42(2):174-9.

* Maillot M, Monsivais P, Drewnowski A. Food pattern modeling shows that the 2010 Dietary Guidelines for sodium and potassium cannot be met simultaneously. Nutr Res. 2013;33(3):188-94.

* Malinauskas BM, Raedeke TD, Aeby VG, et al. Dieting practices, weight perceptions, and body composition: a comparison of normal weight, overweight, and obese college females. Nutr J. 2006;5:11.

* Marcon F, Siniscalchi E, Crebelli R, et al. Diet-related telomere shortening and chromosome stability. Mutagenesis. 2012;27(1):49-57.

* Masternak MM, Bartke A. Growth hormone, inflammation and aging. Pathobiol Aging Age Relat Dis. 2012;2:10.

* Matsumoto M, Kurihara S, Kibe R, et al. Longevity in mice is promoted by probiotic-induced suppression of colonic senescence dependent on upregulation of gut bacterial polyamine production. PLoS One. 2011;6(8):e23652.

* Mattila PT, Pelkonen P, Knuuttila ML. Effects of a long-term dietary xylitol supplementation on collagen content and fluorescence of the skin in aged rats. Gerontology. 2005;51(3):166-9.

* Mays PK, McAnulty RJ, Campa JS, Laurent GJ. Age-related alterations in collagen and total protein metabolism determined in cultured rat dermal fibroblasts: age-related trends parallel those observed in rat skin in vivo. Int J Biochem Cell Biol. 1995;27(9):937-45.

* McCarty MF. Nutraceutical strategies for ameliorating the toxic effects of alcohol. Med Hypotheses. 2013;80(4):456-62.

* McDaniel JC, Massey K, Nicolaou A. Fish oil supplementation alters levels of lipid mediators of inflammation in microenvironment of acute human wounds. Wound Repair Regen. 2011;19(2):189-200.

∗ Milder J, Patel M. Modulation of oxidative stress and mitochondrial function by the ketogenic diet. Epilepsy Res. 2012;100(3):295-303.

∗ Mozaffarian D, Wu JH. Omega-3 fatty acids and cardiovascular disease: effects on risk factors, molecular pathways, and clinical events. J Am Coll Cardiol. 2011;58(20):2047-67.

∗ Nagao K, Yanagita T. Medium-chain fatty acids: functional lipids for the prevention and treatment of the metabolic syndrome. Pharmacol Res. 2010;61(3):208-12.

∗ Nagata C, Nakamura K, Wada K, et al. Association of dietary fat, vegetables and antioxidant micronutrients with skin ageing in Japanese women. Br J Nutr. 2010;103(10):1493-8.

∗ Nanji AA, French SW. Dietary factors and alcoholic cirrhosis. Alcohol Clin Exp Res. 1986;10(3):271-3.

∗ Nettleton JA, Diez-Roux A, Jenny NS, et al. Dietary patterns, food groups, and telomere length in the Multi-Ethnic Study of Atherosclerosis (MESA). Am J Clin Nutr. 2008;88(5):1405-12.

∗ Noguchi O, Takeuchi H, Kubota F, et al. Larger diet-induced thermogenesis and less body fat accumulation in rats fed medium-chain triacylglycerols than in those fed long-chain triacylglycerols. J Nutr Sci Vitaminol (Tokyo). 2002;48(6):524-9.

∗ Noordam R, Gunn DA, Tomlin CC, et al. Cortisol serum levels in familial longevity and perceived age: the Leiden longevity study. Psychoneuroendocrinology. 2012;37(10):1669-75.

∗ Noordam R, Gunn DA, Tomlin CC, et al. High serum glucose levels are associated with a higher perceived age. Age (Dordr). 2013;35(1):189-95.

∗ Noordam R, Gunn DA, Tomlin CC, et al. Serum insulin-like growth factor 1 and facial ageing: high levels associate with reduced skin wrinkling in a cross-sectional study. Br J Dermatol. 2013;168(3):533-8.

* Oh J, Kim JY, Park S, et al. The relationship between insulin-like growth factor-1 and metabolic syndrome, independent of adiponectin. Clin Chim Acta. 2012;413(3-4):506-10.

* Ornish D, Lin J, Daubenmier J, et al. Increased telomerase activity and comprehensive lifestyle changes: a pilot study. Lancet Oncol. 2008;9(11):1048-57.

* Ornish D, Magbanua MJ, Weidner G, et al. Changes in prostate gene expression in men undergoing an intensive nutrition and lifestyle intervention. Proc Natl Acad Sci U S A. 2008;105(24):8369-74.

* Ostman EM, Liljeberg Elmståhl HG, Björck IM. Inconsistency between glycemic and insulinemic responses to regular and fermented milk products. Am J Clin Nutr. 2001;74(1):96-100.

* Ostman E, Granfeldt Y, Persson L, Björck I. Vinegar supplementation lowers glucose and insulin responses and increases satiety after a bread meal in healthy subjects. Eur J Clin Nutr. 2005;59(9):983-8.

* Pageon H. Reaction of glycation and human skin: the effects on the skin and its components, reconstructed skin as a model. Pathol Biol (Paris). 2010;58(3):226-31.

* Pallauf K, Rimbach G. Autophagy, polyphenols and healthy ageing. Ageing Res Rev. 2012;12(1):237-252.

* Park HY, Kim JH, Jung M, et al. A long-standing hyperglycaemic condition impairs skin barrier by accelerating skin ageing process. Exp Dermatol. 2011;20(12):969-74.

* Patere SN, Majumdar AS, Saraf MN. Exacerbation of alcohol-induced oxidative stress in rats by polyunsaturated fatty acids and iron load. Indian J Pharm Sci. 2011;73(2):152-8.

* Pazyar N, Feily A, Kazerouni A. Green tea in dermatology. Skinmed. 2012;10(6):352-5.

✻ Peguet-Navarro J, Dezutter-Dambuyant C, Buetler T, et al. Supplementation with oral probiotic bacteria protects human cutaneous immune homeostasis after UV exposure-double blind, randomized, placebo controlled clinical trial. Eur J Dermatol. 2008;18(5):504-11.

✻ Pelchat ML. Food addiction in humans. J Nutr. 2009;139(3):620-2.

✻ Piccardi N, Manissier P. Nutrition and nutritional supplementation: Impact on skin health and beauty. Dermatoendocrinol. 2009;1(5):271-4.

✻ Pilkington SM, Massey KA, Bennett SP, et al. Randomized controlled trial of oral omega-3 PUFA in solar-simulated radiation-induced suppression of human cutaneous immune responses. Am J Clin Nutr. 2013;97(3):646-52.

✻ Polidori MC, Praticó D, Mangialasche F, et al. High fruit and vegetable intake is positively correlated with antioxidant status and cognitive performance in healthy subjects. J Alzheimers Dis. 2009;17(4):921-7.

✻ Port AM, Ruth MR, Istfan NW. Fructose consumption and cancer: is there a connection? Curr Opin Endocrinol Diabetes Obes. 2012;19(5):367-74.

✻ Popkin BM. Sugary beverages represent a threat to global health. Trends Endocrinol Metab. 2012;23(12):591-3.

✻ Rahman K. Garlic and aging: new insights into an old remedy. Ageing Res Rev. 2003;2(1):39-56.

✻ Ramezani Tehrani F, Moslehi N, Asghari G, et al. Intake of dairy products, calcium, magnesium, and phosphorus in childhood and age at menarche in the Tehran Lipid and Glucose Study. PLoS One. 2013;8(2):e57696.

✻ Reid G, Younes JA, Van der Mei HC, et al. Microbiota restoration: natural and supplemented recovery of human microbial communities. Nat Rev Microbiol. 2011;9(1):27-38.

* Ribaric S. Diet and aging. Oxid Med Cell Longev. 2012;2012:741468.

* Richards MP. A brief review of the archaeological evidence for Palaeolithic and Neolithic subsistence. Eur J Clin Nutr. 2002;56(12):1270-8.

* Rhodes LE, Darby G, Massey KA, et al. Oral green tea catechin metabolites are incorporated into human skin and protect against UV radiation-induced cutaneous inflammation in association with reduced production of pro-inflammatory eicosanoid 12-hydroxyeicosatetraenoic acid. Br J Nutr. 2013;First View:1-10.

* Ros E, Tapsell LC, Sabaté J. Nuts and berries for heart health. Curr Atheroscler Rep. 2010;12(6):397-406.

* Roth LW, Polotsky AJ. Can we live longer by eating less? A review of caloric restriction and longevity. Maturitas. 2012;71(4):315-9.

* Rudman D, Feller AG, Nagraj HS, et al. Effects of human growth hormone in men over 60 years old. N Engl J Med. 1990;323(1):1-6.

* Salvini S, Sera F, Caruso D, et al. Daily consumption of a high-phenol extra-virgin olive oil reduces oxidative DNA damage in postmenopausal women. Br J Nutr. 2006;95(4):742-51.

* Sampey BP, Vanhoose AM, Winfield HM, et al. Cafeteria diet is a robust model of human metabolic syndrome with liver and adipose inflammation: comparison to high-fat diet. Obesity (Silver Spring). 2011;19(6):1109-17.

* Santos FL, Esteves SS, da Costa Pereira A, et al. Systematic review and meta-analysis of clinical trials of the effects of low carbohydrate diets on cardiovascular risk factors. Obes Rev. 2012;13(11):1048-66.

* Sarwar N, Danesh J, Eiriksdottir G, et al. Triglycerides and the risk of coronary heart disease: 10,158 incident cases among 262,525 participants in 29 Western prospective studies. Circulation. 2007;115:450-8.

* Savvas M, Bishop J, Laurent G, et al. Type III collagen content in the skin of postmenopausal women receiving oestradiol and testosterone implants. Br J Obstet Gynaecol. 1993;100(2):154-6.

* Schalkwijk CG, Stehouwer CD, van Hinsbergh VW. Fructose-mediated non-enzymatic glycation: sweet coupling or bad modification. Diabetes Metab Res Rev. 2004;20(5):369-82.

* Schick R, Schusdziarra V. Physiological, pathophysiological and pharmacological aspects of exogenous and endogenous opiates. Clin Physiol Biochem. 1985;3(1):43-60.

* Schinke C, Mo Y, Yu Y, et al. Aberrant DNA methylation in malignant melanoma. Melanoma Res. 2010;20(4):253-65.

* Shen J, Terry MB, Gurvich I, et al. Short telomere length and breast cancer risk: a study in sister sets. Cancer Res. 2007;67(11):5538-44.

* Shotyk W, Krachler M, Chen B. Contamination of Canadian and European bottled waters with antimony from PET containers. J. Environ. Monit. 2006;8:288–92.

* Siri-Tarino PW, Sun Q, Hu FB, Krauss RM. Meta-analysis of prospective cohort studies evaluating the association of saturated fat with cardiovascular disease. Am J Clin Nutr. 2010;91(3):535-46.

* Sisson M. The Primal Blueprint. Ebury Publishing. 2012.

* Soltanian HT, Liu MT, Cash AD, Iglesias RA. Determinants of breast appearance and aging in identical twins. Aesthet Surg J. 2012;32(7):846-60.

* Sonntag WE, Lynch CD, Cefalu WT, et al. J Gerontol A Biol Sci Med Sci. 1999;54(12):B521-38.

* Spector T. Identically Different: Why You Can Change Your Genes. W&N 2012.

* Studd J. Ten reasons to be happy about hormone replacement therapy: a guide for patients. Menopause Int. 2010;16(1):44-6.

* Svendsen L, Rattan SI, Clark BF. Testing garlic for possible anti-ageing effects on long-term growth characteristics, morphology and macromolecular synthesis of human fibroblasts in culture. J Ethnopharmacol. 1994;43(2):125-33.

* Tapsell LC, Hemphill I, Cobiac L, et al. Health benefits of herbs and spices: the past, the present, the future. Med J Aust. 2006;185 (Suppl 4):4-24.

* Thompson PL. J-curve revisited: cardiovascular benefits of moderate alcohol use cannot be dismissed. Med J Aust. 2013;198(8):419-22.

* Thornley S, Tayler R, Sikaris K. Sugar restriction: the evidence for a drug-free intervention to reduce cardiovascular disease risk. Intern Med J. 2012;42(Suppl 5):46-58.

* Tiainen AM, Männistö S, Blomstedt PA, et al. Leukocyte telomere length and its relation to food and nutrient intake in an elderly population. Eur J Clin Nutr. 2012;66(12):1290-4.

* Tucci P. Caloric restriction: is mammalian life extension linked to p53? Aging (Albany NY). 2012;4(8):525-34.

* Valtin H. "Drink at least eight glasses of water a day." Really? Is there scientific evidence for "8 x 8"? Am J Physiol Regul Integr Comp Physiol. 2002;283(5):R993-1004.

* Van Grinsven HJ, Rabl A, de Kok TM. Estimation of incidence and social cost of colon cancer due to nitrate in drinking water in the EU: a tentative cost-benefit assessment. Environ Health. 2010;9:58.

* Vazzana N, Ranalli P, Cuccurullo C, Davì G. Diabetes mellitus and thrombosis. Thromb Res. 2012;129(3):371-7.

* Vellai T. Autophagy genes and ageing. Cell Death Differ. 2009;16(1):94-102.

* Ventegodt S, Merrick J. Dean Ornish should receive the Nobel prize in medicine. Int J Adolesc Med Health. 2012;24(2):97-8.

* Verdier-Sévrain S. Effect of estrogens on skin aging and the potential role of selective estrogen receptor modulators. Climacteric. 2007;10(4):289-97.

* Vinson JA, Cai Y. Nuts, especially walnuts, have both antioxidant quantity and efficacy and exhibit significant potential health benefits. Food Funct. 2012;3(2):134-40.

* Vitale G, Brugts MP, Ogliari G, et al. Low circulating IGF-I bioactivity is associated with human longevity: findings in centenarians' offspring. Aging (Albany NY). 2012;4(9):580-9.

* Volek JS, Phinney SD. The Art and Science of Low Carbohydrate Living: An Expert Guide to Making the Life-Saving Benefits of Carbohydrate Restriction Sustainable and Enjoyable. Beyond Obesity LLC. 2011.

* Voon PT, Ng TK, Lee VK, Nesaretnam K. Diets high in palmitic acid (16:0), lauric and myristic acids (12:0 + 14:0), or oleic acid (18:1) do not alter postprandial or fasting plasma homocysteine and inflammatory markers in healthy Malaysian adults. Am J Clin Nutr. 2011;94(6):1451-7.

* Vitale G, Brugts MP, Ogliari G, et al. Low circulating IGF-I bioactivity is associated with human longevity: findings in centenarians' offspring. Aging (Albany NY). 2012;4(9):580-9.

* Von Mühlen D, Laughlin GA, Kritz-Silverstein D, Barrett-Connor E. The Dehydroepiandrosterone And WellNess (DAWN) study: research design and methods. Contemp Clin Trials. 2007;28(2):153-68.

* Wang L, Hao Q, Wang YD, et al. Protective effects of dehydroepiandrosterone on atherosclerosis in ovariectomized rabbits via alleviating inflammatory injury in endothelial cells. Atherosclerosis. 2011;214(1):47-57.

* Wentzensen IM, Mirabello L, Pfeiffer RM, Savage SA. The association of telomere length and cancer: a meta-analysis. Cancer Epidemiol Biomarkers Prev. 2011;20(6):1238-50.

* Whitehead RD, Ozakinci G, Perrett DI. Attractive skin coloration: harnessing sexual selection to improve diet and health. Evol Psychol. 2012;10(5):842-54.

* Wijsman CA, Rozing MP, Streefland TC, et al. Familial longevity is marked by enhanced insulin sensitivity. Aging Cell. 2011;10(1):114-21.

* Wilcox G. Insulin and Insulin Resistance. Clin Biochem Rev. 2005;26(2): 19-39.

* Williams S, Tamburic S, Lally C. Eating chocolate can significantly protect the skin from UV light. J Cosmet Dermatol. 2009;8(3):169-73.

* Xu Q, Parks CG, DeRoo LA, et al. Multivitamin use and telomere length in women. Am J Clin Nutr. 2009;89(6):1857-63.

* Yang Q, Liu T, Kuklina EV, et al. Sodium and potassium intake and mortality among US adults: prospective data from the Third National Health and Nutrition Examination Survey. Arch Intern Med. 2011;171(13):1183-91.

* Zouboulis ChC. [Intrinsic skin aging. A critical appraisal of the role of hormones]. Hautarzt. 2003;54(9):825-32.

* Zou S, Carey JR, Liedo P, et al. Prolongevity effects of a botanical with oregano and cranberry extracts in Mexican fruit flies: examining interactions of diet restriction and age. Age (Dordr). 2012;34(2):269-79.